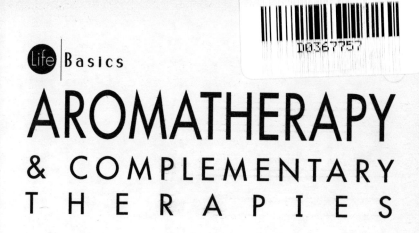

Life|Basics

AROMATHERAPY
& COMPLEMENTARY
THERAPIES

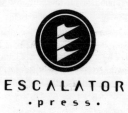

ESCALATOR
• press •

Published through special arrangement with
Strathearn Books Ltd

This edition published by Escalator Press
Distributed by Stewart House Publishing Inc.
Etobicoke, Canada

© 2001 Geddes & Grosset,
David Dale House, New Lanark, ML11 9DJ, Scotland

First published in this edition 2002

Cover image courtesy of PhotoDisc, Inc.

ISBN 1 55366 278 4

Printed and bound in Europe

Contents

Warning

The following essential oils should *never* be used under any circumstances as they are extremely poisonous.

bitter almond	sassafras
boldo leaf	savin
calamus	southernwood
horseradish	tansy
jaborandi leaf	thuja
mugwort	wintergreen
mustard	wormwood
pennyroyal	wormseed
rue	yellow camphor

Do not undertake any course of treatment without the advice of your doctor.

Never stop taking medication without the agreement of your doctor.

Some essential oils, when used inappropriately can be highly toxic. Some essential oils are unsuitable for use at home. Consult a professional aromatherapist before undertaking any course of treatment with essential oils.

Do not use essential oils in pregnancy, or on babies and young children, without the advice of a trained aromatherapist.

Some medical conditions contraindicate the use of certain essential oils and/or massage.

Do not ingest essential oils.

Do not use essential oils in the eyes.

Do not use essential oils undiluted on the skin unless otherwise indicated.

If using homeopathy or herbal medicine in conjunction with aromatherapy, seek the advice of the relevant practitioner as well as the aromatherapist.

What is Aromatherapy?

Aromatherapy is the term used for a form of therapy that makes use of the essential oils of a large number of aromatic plants, shrubs and trees. The oils extracted from the plants can be used in a variety of different ways, for the treatment of both medical and psychological conditions, for cosmetic purposes, or simply for pleasure. Essential oils can affect both the physical and mental state of an individual, and scientific research continues into the precise manner in which the oils take effect.

Aromatherapy has been practised for a very long time. Its rise in popularity in recent years has partially contributed to its being labelled by some people as a New Age therapy, but this is hardly an appropriate way to describe a use of plants and essential oils that has a history of several hundreds of years. Moreover, it is unfortunate that the New Age label brings with it more than a little prejudice. New Age is a term that sceptics tend to use in a derogatory sense, as if New Age equates with 'mumbo-jumbo'. What the sceptics will be unlikely to admit is that they, like all of us, probably indulge in some sort of aromatherapy in their everyday lives, whether they realize it or not.

Qualified aromatherapists require a great deal of knowledge and expertise to enable them to practise. Their skills can be invaluable in the treatment of many ailments, whether these ailments require additional conventional medical treatment or not. Sometimes aromatherapy will be used as a treatment. It has many applications in the treatment of a wide variety of ailments, some relatively minor, others of a more serious nature. As research into the subject continues, so the possibilities of aromatherapy expand. At other times, aromatherapy will be used as a palliative. Where it is used properly, it can do much to make a person feel better in himself or herself, even if it cannot effect a cure.

We are often our own aromatherapists in a sense. Certain smells can make us feel good, so, for example, we choose the bath oil with the smell that soothes our spirits. Certain essential oils can ease aching muscles and relax a tired body. We can find such oils in some 'conventional' soaps, bath oils, skin creams and lotions. When we use such things, we are, in a sense, practising aromatherapy, even if we do not call it that. When we have a cold, we can make use of eucalyptus oil – a few drops on a handkerchief can be sniffed from time to time to clear a stuffy nose. Teenagers can use tea-tree oil, or preparations containing tea-tree oil, to treat spots. It is all aromatherapy. When we sniff the flowers that we are choosing for a bouquet, enjoy the fresh scent of pine on a forest walk or pick fresh herbs from the garden for cooking – enjoying the pungent aroma that is given off by the bruised leaves of the plants – we are experiencing aromatherapy.

People have had more detailed knowledge of the secrets of the treatment now called aromatherapy for many centuries. Long before medical science was able to call upon the services of chemists, people were using extracts from plants and trees in herbal medicine, in the prevention of disease and in religious and public ceremonies all over the world.

As medical science has progressed, there has been a certain tendency for the real proven benefits of plant-based medicine to be overlooked in favour of artificial substitutes. In spite of the fact that some of the most commonly used drugs, such as digoxin, were developed from plants and are still made from plant derivatives, many people are sceptical about herbal medicine and even more dubious about the therapeutic possibilities of aromatherapy, which, after all, is also plant-based. Perhaps it is because doctors do not study aromatherapy at medical school. Perhaps it is because aromatherapy treatments do not come in the same ready-prepared and measured doses as conventional medical treatments – pills to be swallowed or fluids to be injected. There is certainly a measure of doubt in the minds of some people that something that is applied externally, as essential oils are for the most part, can have a real effect on the internal workings of the body. Nonetheless, those who take the time to find out more about aromatherapy and to try it for themselves are rarely disappointed. Aromatherapy is age-old rather than New Age, and it has many benefits to offer.

The holistic approach

Aromatherapy is a holistic form of treatment. A skilled aromatherapist will always take a patient's history in some detail. The aim is to treat the whole person rather than the symptoms alone. This approach has three benefits. Firstly, it can help patients, perhaps for the first time in years, to take a good look at themselves, their lifestyles, their states of mind, including attitudes to themselves and to their lives, and the mental and physical demands that are made on them. (Many people pay no attention to their own health until something goes wrong.) Thus made more self-aware, patients are given the chance to see beyond their symptoms, to increase their self-knowledge and to look towards ways of improving their general mental and physical wellbeing, which in turn will encourage the body to increase its ability to heal itself and combat further disease.

The second benefit of the holistic approach is that it enables the aromatherapist to look more closely at the patient, rather than just at any specific problems with which the patient has presented, to try to establish better the root causes of any ailments and thus to treat the patient rather than the symptoms alone. If the symptoms of any disease are alleviated but the cause of these symptoms is not tackled the problem is likely to return. For example, if a patient presents with a complaint that is stress-related, the aromatherapist should be able not only to help the patient to relieve the immediate symptoms but also to work with the patient to tackle the stress itself, providing both relaxing treatment and beneficial advice.

Thirdly and lastly, the holistic approach is undoubtedly beneficial simply because it takes time. There can be little doubt of the benefits of having someone taking time to listen and to care, especially in today's world, when life seems to pass at such breakneck speed.

Aromatherapy is not a substitute for conventional medicine. No aromatherapist would claim that it is. Aromatherapists are well aware that essential oils can treat a whole catalogue of problems and also have the potential to be used in the treatment of many more, but they are not in the business of producing 'miracle' cures.

What aromatherapy does offer is a form of treatment that

can do much to improve a person's general state of mental and physical wellbeing, to promote a state of balance within mind and body which will enable the individual to cope better with illness, stress and fatigue – in short, to help the body to heal itself. Aromatherapy can be used in conjunction with conventional medical treatment quite successfully, provided that both doctor and aromatherapist are aware of each other's roles in the patient's care. In many circumstances aromatherapy can offer an effective alternative to conventional forms of therapy for many physical and mental problems, an alternative that is pleasant to undergo and is free from undesirable side effects.

Caution

A word of warning: aromatherapy, practised responsibly at home, is safe and effective for the treatment of many minor complaints – muscular aches and pains, colds and 'flu, cuts, scrapes and spots, etc – but **the diagnosis and treatment of serious problems, or problems that you suspect might be serious, should always be left to the experts**. It is foolhardy and dangerous to 'play doctor'.

The benefits of massage

Aromatherapists use massage as their main method for the application of essential oils. Usually, a full body massage will be given, using oils that have been selected as being most appropriate for the patient. Specific areas of discomfort can also be given particular attention. Massage is an effective means of ensuring that the essential oils, which have been diluted in carrier oils, are penetrating the patient's skin. As a proportion of the volatile oils vaporizes with the heat of the patient's skin, extra benefit will be gained from inhaling them.

The use of essential oils in massage, which combines application and therapeutic touch, can be beneficial in many ways.

We all, from birth onwards, appreciate the comfort that the touch of another human being can bring. When a young baby cries, its mother instinctively picks it up and soothes it in her arms, stroking and patting to bring reassurance and to help restore calm. When a child falls, the sore knee might be kissed or gently rubbed 'all better'. As we grow older, touch remains the most instinctive means of showing care and concern and offering comfort, from the sympathetic hand on another's shoulder to a warm, soothing hug. When we feel pain in our muscles, it comes naturally to us to hold, or rub, the affected part. In this way, we act as our own comforters. We are also, by giving heat and gentle friction to the area that is painful, dilating blood vessels and improving circulation to accelerate healing. (In some cases, where there is acute inflammation present, the application of heat is inappropriate, but if this is so then we are unlikely to want to touch the affected area. It will be too painful.) Massage also stimulates the lymphatic system, helping the body to rid itself of toxins.

Massage is enjoyable. It is possibly the single most pleasurable form of therapy. It relaxes the body, soothes the soul and calms the troubled mind. It is an invaluable weapon in the war against stress and can uplift the spirits of those who feel tired and depressed. Aside from the benefits that can be gained from the appropriate selection of essential oils for use in massage, the worth of the act itself can never be underestimated.

Massage can also be carried out between sexual partners, when it can be enjoyable for both the masseur and the one who is being massaged. Of course, it can be used erotically and can do much to enhance a loving sexual relationship, but massage does not have to be erotic to be pleasurable and sensual and to bring a couple closer together.

Many members of the medical professions are now appreciating the value of touch and massage. Mothers will often be advised by midwives that a gentle massage with sweet almond oil can be an effective way to soothe a fretful or 'jumpy' baby and to help cement the bond between mother and child. Babies isolated in incubators fare better when they are reassured with gentle stroking and a soothing touch. Many general practitioners are now quite willing to suggest aromatherapy and massage to patients suffering from the effects of stress. The nursing profession has also become increasingly aware of the benefits of massage and aromatherapy and its applications in their profession.

Different massage techniques can be used with different effects – details are given in the chapter on massage *(see* page 168) – but it is perfectly reasonable to state that unless the subject suffers from a condition that renders massage inadvisable, the practice of basic, gentle massage is quite safe and as long as the subject finds it enjoyable, specific health benefits apart, he or she will undoubtedly gain from it. In a world where everything moves so fast, where everybody feels the pressure to work harder and faster and longer, many people get precious few moments when they can take time, take stock and take care of themselves. The practice of massage might seem like an indulgence, but it is an indulgence that is easily justified. Unlike some of the other means by which people choose to seek pleasure and relaxation, such as alcohol, drugs and cigarettes, massage is harmless, beneficial to body and spirit, caring and bonding. We have every right to enjoy it.

Aromatherapy through time

Simple, everyday uses of many aromatic plants, such as parsley or aniseed to freshen breath, or lavender to soothe and rosemary to lift the spirits, go back many hundreds of years. The use of aromatic plants in herbal medicine is well documented and centuries old. Aromatherapy is derived from herbal medicine, using as it does a vital constituent part of the aromatic plant, i.e., the essential oil. Essential oils, like the plants from which they are extracted, also have a history of use that goes back centuries.

Many ancient civilizations appreciated the properties of the essential oils of certain plants. The Greeks, Romans, Chinese, Egyptians, Arabs, Persians and the aboriginal people of Australia, India and Africa are all known to have used essential oils as perfumes, medicines, incenses and in other ways for many hundreds of years.

Much of what we know of the ancient Egyptian people has come from the recovery of treasures and writings from the ancient tombs of the wealthy and prominent members of their society, tombs so beautifully and carefully constructed that they stand to this day. The tombs also contained the remains of the dead, meticulously preserved by the process of embalming, a process that made extensive use of essential oils such as cedarwood and myrrh. The Egyptians also used aromatic plants medicinally and for making perfumes –

Cleopatra was not alone in knowing that perfumes made from certain plants had an aphrodisiac effect!

The antiseptic properties of the essential oils of certain plants were appreciated by the ancient Romans and Greeks among others. The Greeks used thyme, for example, as a fumigating agent, burning sprigs of the plant in areas where disease was present in order to prevent further spread. On the other side of the world, the Aboriginal people of Australia used eucalyptus, another strongly antiseptic plant, in much the same way. Hippocrates, the Greek physician who lived in the first century BC and whose writings and teachings showed him to be a genius of his time in the practice of medicine and surgery, made use of aromatics and of massage in his practice. Like the ancient Egyptians, the Greeks and Romans also made extensive use of aromatic plants in making perfumes and ointments, as did the Syrians and the Indian and Arab peoples.

Ayurvedic medicine, practised in India for more than three thousand years, has much in common with aromatherapy as we know it today as it uses aromatic oils in massage as one of its principal elements.

We know of the use of myrrh from various sources, but the most familiar source to most of us will be the Bible, which contains many references to precious oils and ointments. In the New Testament it is written that myrrh was brought to the infant Jesus as a birth gift by one of the three wise men from the East. Myrrh was prized in various cultures, not only as a perfume and incense ingredient but also as a disinfecting and healing agent.

Frankincense was another gift to the Christ child, another much valued ingredient of incense and medicinal oil that was used in many countries, including Arabia, China, ancient Rome and Egypt.

Basil is another particular example of a plant that has been used by many cultures for hundreds of years, for its antiseptic properties, its digestive uses and its flavour. It was used along with myrrh and incense by the ancient Egyptians for embalming. Basil oil has been used medicinally for many hundreds of years in Eastern cultures, and in ancient Rome and Greece it was used for bathing and antisepsis. In India, it has religious significance for Hindus, who believe it to be sacred to the god Krishna.

As centuries passed and people travelled farther, different cultures imparted their secrets to one another and knowledge spread. The uses of aromatic plants and the art of distillation to make them yield their precious essential oils became known far and wide across the world. Aromatic plants and trees also spread from country to country, making it possible for people from countries where the plants were not indigenous to access their potential more easily. The crusaders in the twelfth century did much to spread the knowledge of the art of perfumery in Europe. In the Middle Ages perfumes imported from other countries became increasingly used in Great Britain. In times when personal hygiene was virtually non-existent and people rarely washed, the exotic perfumes brought from countries afar were much appreciated for their ability to mask other, less pleasant odours. The disinfectant properties of aromatic plants were also appreciated and brought into use in times of typhoid, cholera and plague.

Through the centuries, knowledge of herbal medicine increased and, in conjunction with this, knowledge of many of the uses of essential oils distilled from aromatic plants. Herbs formed the basis of the doctors' medical armoury. Essential oils were used and appreciated by two distinct professions: the medical profession and the perfumers. Each had its own band of scientists working to analyse the properties of the essential oils and ways in which to use them. The perfume and cosmetics industry grew increasingly sophisticated, and the chemists working in the field of medicine steadily worked on analysis of the chemical constituents of essential oils, identifying them and striving to replicate them in artificial preparations.

Gradually, through the eighteenth century and beyond, medical science moved on in this direction and, increasingly, doctors and chemists began to make use of chemical alternatives to traditional medicines. Whereas herbal medicine had been quite readily accessible to the average person, the new medicine was not. Doctors and scientists were now in charge. Gradually, the average man in the street came to rely more upon the professional 'medicine men' than upon the knowledge that had been passed down through families for years. Herbal medicine was now old-fashioned. Indeed, by the twentieth century, it was viewed by many with suspicion.

The specific art of aromatherapy as it is practised nowadays owes a great deal to the work of the French. The first of these were Chamberland, Meunier and Cadeac who carried out research towards the end of the nineteenth century on the efficacy of essential oils as antibacterial agents. Then in the late 1920s a French chemist called Rene Gattefosse coined the term 'aromatherapy' for the first time. He had discovered, quite by accident, that lavender oil seemed to have a beneficial effect on burnt skin. He burnt his hand while working in his laboratory and instinctively applied the nearest liquid that was to hand to ease the pain. It was lavender oil. He noticed that his hand healed remarkably quickly and that scarring was minimized. This prompted him to carry out further tests on other essential oils, and he was intrigued to find the range of medicinal properties of these oils, both in the prevention and treatment of disease. He predicted that much could be achieved if their potential was realized.

In the 1940s, another Frenchman, called Jean Valnet, a surgeon who took inspiration from Gattefosse's work, became absorbed in the subject and carried out a great deal of research of his own. He had already discovered, in the course of his work as a military surgeon during the Second World War, that essential oils were invaluable for their antiseptic properties and in the treatment of wounds. He also came to realize that essential oils worked not only on the body but also on the psychological state of the individual. He became intrigued by the possibilities that this held for the treatment of some kinds of psychiatric illness. Further work with aromatics led to the publication of a book in the 1960s, entitled *Aromatherapie*. Many regard Gattefosse and Valnet as the 'fathers' of modern aromatherapy.

Another very important figure in the field, contemporary with Valnet, was Marguerite Maury, an Austrian chemist and beautician who did much to establish aromatherapy in Europe both for its cosmetic and for its medicinal applications. She was particularly interested in using essential oils in massage.

Interest in aromatherapy has been growing over time. It is true, however, that most people are still completely reliant on over-the-counter cosmetics and medical preparations that have been purchased at a pharmacy or prescribed by a doctor and consequently know little of the true potential of plants and their essences. Nevertheless, interest continues to grow to such an extent that large companies have spotted the potential in the market and now essential oils and aromatherapy products can be purchased in most high street pharmacies. Although for the most part these products are intended for cosmetic use, it is now easy for the individual to find relevant literature for information on the subject and on the essential oils for personal use. Aromatherapists worldwide have established professional organizations with their own training courses and qualifications, both for those people who wish to practise professionally and for those whose interest remains at a personal level.

We have every reason to be grateful to the medical and pharmacological sciences and the enormous advances that have been made in these fields, but it would be a pity to overlook the enormous benefits that 'alternative' – and ancient – therapies, such as aromatherapy, can bring. The upsurge of interest in aromatherapy in recent times has already gone some way to redress the balance. More and more people are beginning to see its value, both when used in conjunction with conventional medicine and sometimes as a useful and often more pleasant alternative to drug treatment.

Scientific research into the precise effects of individual oils and their chemical elements is continuing and there is much to hope for – the full potential of aromatherapy is yet to be realized.

The nature of essential oils
Essential oils are all extractions from living plants and trees,

whether cultivated or wild. It is the essential oil that gives the plant its distinctive smell and, if the plant is edible, its flavour. Essential oils are extracted from different parts of different plants. Some plants, such as jasmine, yield their oils from the flower; others, such as rosemary, do so from the leaves. Other kinds of plant contain essential oils in their seeds, in their roots or, in the case of some trees, in the wood or bark. Essential oils can also be extracted from some aromatic grasses. There are currently more than two hundred plants and trees from which essential oils are extracted, although not all these essential oils can be used therapeutically.

In some plants, the essential oil is contained in microscopic quantities whilst in others there are more generous amounts. Similarly, some essential oils are much easier to extract than others. Jasmine, a flower much prized by the perfume industry for its heady scent, yields, with reluctance, notoriously small quantities of its precious essential oil. For every ounce of oil that is produced, one thousand times that weight of flowers must be used. On the other hand, three different essential oils can be extracted from citrus fruit trees: the flowers, the leaves and the skin of the fruit all contain essential oils. It is particularly easy to extract the oil from the skin and pith of the fruit. They are squeezed by hand or (much more frequently nowadays) in a mechanical press to express the vital juices.

The herbs that are particularly enjoyable to touch in the garden, giving off a waft of aroma when their leaves are rubbed between the fingers, release minute quantities of their essential oils into the atmosphere and onto the skin. Some of these oils have particularly lingering perfumes. Lavender oil is like this. Old-fashioned lavender bags, filled with dried lavender flower heads, make long-lasting and effective drawer fresheners.

Essential oils are volatile substances that evaporate easily when heated. They all contain a complex combination of many different chemicals which give them their individual qualities and effects. Terpenes are an important component in the citrus oils, for example. It is the terpene content in these oils that makes them prone to more rapid oxidization and deterioration than some other essential oils. Most essential oils are high in alcohols, which give them their antiseptic properties. Esters, another group of chemicals found in many essential oils, have a sedative effect. Essential oils that contain high proportions of phenols will have anti-bacterial qualities. The chemical make-up of each herb is also dependent to some extent on the place where it has been cultivated. Thus two samples of the same herb, grown in different places and under different conditions, can produce oils that have a slightly different chemical make-up.

Not all essential oils are suitable for therapeutic use. Some are highly toxic. It is interesting to note that the essential oils of certain herbs and spices that are widely used for culinary purposes fall into this category. For example, mustard is considered an essential condiment in kitchens all over the world. The essential oil extracted from mustard seeds, however, is extremely toxic. It has no therapeutic use whatsoever. The leaves of the herb chervil make a refreshing addition to salads, and the juice obtained fresh from the leaves is used in herbal medicine for its healing properties, but essential oil of chervil is toxic, an irritant and a possible carcinogen.

Some essential oils are free-flowing liquids, whilst others

are more viscous and some are solid or semi-solid until heated. Essential oils dissolve easily in alcohol and oil but not in water. The volatility of essential oils, their swift evaporation when exposed to heat, is a property that is exploited both in the extraction processes and in the therapeutic use of the oils.

Essential oils are very concentrated and the vast majority of them irritate the skin when used neat. Some are quite toxic unless well diluted. Used in appropriate dilution, however, they all have their own distinct therapeutic qualities, and many of them can be used and enjoyed quite safely and with beneficial effects in a domestic environment by 'lay' people.

CAUTION:

- As a general rule, essential oils should never be applied neat to the skin. Exceptions to this rule are tea tree and lavender.
- Essential oils are flammable – extremely so. If you use them in a burner, put a few drops in water – not oil – in the bowl of the burner and allow the perfume to enter the atmosphere through evaporation.
- Although some practitioners will occasionally prescribe essential oils by mouth, this is the exception rather then the rule. **When using essential oils at home, use them for external application only.** Unless they have been specifically prescribed by a qualified person, it should be assumed that they are not safe to be ingested. Some essential oils are very toxic indeed if swallowed. Some oils have benefits in the treatment of certain oral ailments, when used as a mouthwash or gargle in recommended dilution, but even so should **never** be swallowed.

- If you are storing essential oils at home, make sure that they are kept well out of the reach of children.
- Always seek the advice of a trained aromatherapist if you wish to use essential oils during pregnancy or on babies and young children.
- If using homeopathy or herbal medicine seek the advice of the relevant practitioner as well as that of an aromatherapist
- Some medical conditions contraindicate the use of certain essential oils and/or massage. If you suffer from any kind of medical condition always check with your doctor first and always consult a trained aromatherapist before you use essential oils.

The Extraction of Essential Oils

Steam distillation

Essential oils are extracted from different parts of different plants. The most common method of oil extraction is by steam distillation. In countries where the source plants are grown, stills are more often than not kept very close to the cultivation areas to ensure the optimum freshness of the plants used for distillation. The appropriate part of the plant – seeds, leaves, stems, flowers or a combination of more than one of these – is compacted into the first container in the still. Steam is then passed through the still and the essential oil evaporates with the heat of the steam. The evaporated essential oil rises and passes, with the steam, through a condenser and into a collecting vessel where cooling takes place. When the essential oil and water are cooled, the oil will separate from the water and can be siphoned off the top.

Some plants, such as jasmine, do not respond well to steam distillation as the heat is too intense to preserve the odour. Two different methods of extraction are used in cases such as this. What is produced by these processes is not, strictly speaking, an essential oil but an absolute.

Enfleurage

The first process, enfleurage, is still practised by some perfumeries in France, sometimes only for demonstration purposes for the benefit of visiting tourists, but it is more or less obsolete elsewhere. It is labour-intensive and extremely slow, but it produces a very high quality jasmine absolute that is strong and pure. The jasmine flowers are spread out by hand on glass trays containing special fat. The trays are then stacked up and left lying to give the oil time to penetrate the fat. The process is then repeated, the used flowers being lifted off and replaced with fresh ones, until the fat is absolutely saturated with essential oil. The saturated fat is known as a pomade. When the pomade is ready it is then processed with alcohol to separate the jasmine absolute. The residue fat in the enfleurage process need not be wasted. It retains some of the odour of the jasmine and can be used for soap manufacture.

Solvent extraction

The second method of extracting jasmine absolute is by solvent extraction; some other plants are also processed in a similar way.

The flowers (or relevant parts of the plant) are macerated and mixed in a container with a solvent such as hexane. The extract is then heated to vaporize the solvent that now contains the essential oil and plant waxes. When the solvent has evaporated, what remains is known as a concrete, roughly half absolute and half plant wax.

After cooling, further processing of the concrete with alcohol separates the absolute from the wax.

Resinoids are also produced by solvent extraction from gums and resinous materials. Some resinoids can be further processed with alcohol to produce an absolute.

Carbon dioxide extraction

Carbon dioxide extraction is a relatively new process compared to the others but may become a method preferred to solvent extraction over time. There is some concern about the amounts of solvent that remain in the concretes and absolutes after solvent extraction and the use of carbon dioxide avoids this problem.

Essential Oils at Work

Essential oils work on two distinct levels, the psychological and the physical.

Imagine some of your favourite aromas. How do they make you feel? Certain smells can trigger happy memories of places or people, taking you back to early childhood, to the kitchen at home, perhaps, or to a particular person, such as your mother. Some smells will make you think of a certain time of year – the freshness of spring or the sun-baked days of summer. Other smells that you find enjoyable might be harder to explain – they simply make you feel good. If you are trying to sell your house, the estate agent may well tell you to put a pot of coffee on the stove before prospective buyers come to view, or make some bread or cakes to fill the house with the scent of fresh baking. Smell is a primitive and powerful sense. Not only can it alert us to danger (think of the odour of meat that has gone bad or the smell of a gas leak), it can also trigger memories, alter our moods and either attract us to, or put us off, potential mates. Recent research has shown that human beings have not yet become so sophisticated that the sense of smell has become irrelevant in the process of sexual attraction. No matter how beautiful, intelligent and witty you might be, the object of your heart's desire will still be affected by your own, very individual smell.

The fragrant essential oils of many plants can have quite a powerful effect on the mind, altering mood quite noticeably when they are inhaled. This is what makes aromatherapy particularly useful in the treatment of mood disturbances such as depression and anxiety and the consequent effects these problems have on the individual's ability to function properly. Some oils will have a definite sedative, calming effect, whilst others are useful for their stimulant properties, increasing mental and physical energy. Certain oils are particularly good at helping to focus the mind; such oils are often burned in incense, as an aid to meditation. Some oils will stimulate sexual appetites and can be used as aphrodisiacs.

It is still something of a mystery as to how the smells of essential oils can affect emotion and mood so profoundly. The odours of the oils are taken up by receptor cells within the nasal cavity which are connected, via the olfactory nerve, to the limbic system in the brain – the part of the brain that controls emotion and memory. Whether the response of the brain is entirely because of the particular chemical make-up of the oils is uncertain, but the brain is stimulated by the smells to release certain neurochemicals into the bloodstream. Some neurochemicals, such as serotonin, promote relaxation and can induce sleep while others have a stimulating effect. Endorphins are another group of chemicals that can be produced in response to essential oil odours. These are opiate-like substances that inhibit pain and induce a feeling of wellbeing. They are, in short, 'feel-good' chemicals.

On a purely physiological level, different essential oils, according to their individual chemical make-up, will each have their own specific effects on the internal workings of the body.

There are three ways by which essential oils can enter the

body. The first of these is by inhalation, which allows for the oil molecules to enter the body through the tiny capillaries supplying the respiratory organs.

Essential oils can also be absorbed into the body by skin absorption – by bathing in hot water to which oils have been added, by applying essential oils in topical preparations or in compresses, and by massage.

The third means by which essential oils can enter the body is by ingestion. Some qualified aromatherapists will prescribe the use of some essential oils in this way, but on the whole massage is the preferred method of treatment. **Ingestion of essential oils is potentially very dangerous and should never be tried in the home.**

One property that many essential oils have in common is the ability to stimulate the body's immune system, that is, to encourage the body to heal itself. Antiseptic and bactericidal properties are also common to most essential oils eucalyptus oil and tea-tree oil being particularly useful in this respect. Many oils (tea-tree oil falls into this category too) have anti-viral and/or fungicidal properties.

Antibiotics have for many years been an invaluable weapon in the war against many diseases, but overuse has led to an increase in antibiotic-resistant strains of bacteria. Antibiotics also kill off many other, harmless and/or beneficial bacteria, leading to problems such as *Candida albicans*, or thrush, and they can have unpleasant side effects. When suffering from a relatively minor infection that is likely to respond well to treatment with essential oils, it makes a lot of sense to choose this option rather than resorting to antibiotics.

Massage

This is the main method of treatment used by qualified aromatherapists. Massage allows for a combination of the beneficial effects of the absorption of essential oils through the skin and those of therapeutic massage; as the therapist's hands work on the patient's body, circulation and lymphatic drainage will be stimulated and the patient's muscles will relax. At the same time, helped by the heat caused by the friction of the therapist's hands on the patient's body, the oil molecules can enter the body through the skin and will start to take effect on the patient. The patient will gain further benefit as he or she breathes in the fragrance. While not all the oils that are used by aromatherapists in practice are recommended for use in the home, there is nonetheless a wide variety of essential oils that can be used perfectly safely by people who lack the aromatherapists' expertise but want to derive some benefit and pleasure from home massage. Massage techniques are detailed in the relevant chapter (*see* page 168). Essential oils for massage can be diluted in a base oil, either singly or blended with one or two other harmonizing, synergistic, oils. Base oils suitable for aromatherapy include almond oil, avocado oil, jojoba oil, and wheatgerm oil – *see* Selecting and Using Base Oils, page 53. Doubtless you will have your own preferences, but each has its own qualities; avocado, for example, is beneficial to dry skin. Try to establish that the base oil you intend to use has been cold-pressed and preferably is organic and thus as pure and chemical-free as possible. When it comes to the dilution quantities, 1–3 per cent essential oil to base oil is generally a safe option, but if you have any doubts, you can check with an aromatherapist.

Inhalation

Steam inhalation is used mostly for the treatment of respiratory disorders. To prepare, fill a fairly large bowl with very hot water and add a few drops of the essential oil, or oils, of choice. Drape a towel over your head and 'tent' it all round the bowl then breathe in the scented steam deeply. Continue treatment for a few minutes, but stop if you feel too hot. Place the bowl on a surface at a height that does not require you to bend over it. Raising your head suddenly, especially if you have been bending over, might cause dizziness. Steam inhalation is beneficial to respiratory ailments in two ways. Firstly, the steam moistens the airways and helps to loosen mucus and clear blocked sinuses. Secondly, the essential oil vapours will enter the bloodstream rapidly and work their own individual 'magic', whether this is to promote expectoration or fight off infection.

Dry inhalation is also beneficial with certain aromatic oils and can be useful in the treatment of asthmatics, whose lungs may be irritated by steam inhalation. A few drops of essential oil can be applied to a handkerchief that is then held a few inches under the patient's nose as he or she breathes in. Alternatively, a few drops can be placed on the pillow (away from the eyes) at bedtime. Eucalyptus oil is a favourite for use in dry inhalation to ease the discomfort of blocked noses. Lavender oil on the pillow will help promote restful sleep.

If you are treating oily skin with aromatic steam, it is pleasant to finish treatment with a refreshing splash of rose water, which will tone the skin. Steam treatment is not recommended if you suffer from thread veins or if you have any inflammatory skin condition.

Steam facial

A steam facial, taken in much the same way as a steam inhalation, can be a very effective way of opening the pores and cleansing the skin, particularly skin that is prone to oiliness and spots. There are several essential oils that can be used in this way. It is pleasant and refreshing to finish off the treatment with a splash of rose water.

CAUTION

Do not use steam facials if you have broken veins or very sensitive skin.

Bathing

Aromatic bathing is a wonderful way to treat yourself and do yourself some good at the same time. Bathing with essential oils allows for the oil to be absorbed firstly through the skin and secondly, as the oils evaporate in the steam from the bath, through inhalation of the fragrant steamy atmosphere in the bathroom. This form of treatment has the advantage that, unlike massage, it can be done without the help of another person.

Run a hot bath with the door and windows closed and add a few drops (3–10, depending on the oil or oils of choice) of essential oil into the water. Make sure that the oil is thoroughly dispersed in the water to avoid the possibility of concentrated amounts of oil coming into contact with the skin. Prolonged and frequent use of essential oils can damage the surface of some baths; make sure the bath is thoroughly cleaned out afterwards. To avoid problems with sensitive skin, and also to preserve your bath, dilute the essential oil in a base oil before you add it to the bath. You can also dilute the essential oil in milk.

Choose your essential oil or oils according to the desired effect you wish to achieve – rosemary to revive your flagging spirits, perhaps, or chamomile to set you up for a good night's sleep. Take all the time you need – lie back in the water and breathe deeply – an aromatic bath should be a very pleasurable experience.

NOTE

Don't use soaps, bath oils or shampoos in an aromatic bath. If you want to clean yourself with soap, or wash your hair, do this beforehand – have a quick shower or wash before you run your aromatic bath.

An aromatic footbath is also a soothing and refreshing way of treating tired, aching feet and will benefit not only your feet but also your whole body. If you only have a shower at home, treat yourself to a footbath from time to time. Lavender, peppermint and rosemary are particularly beneficial at the end of a long day. Footbaths can also help to warm cold feet, and the addition of appropriate oils will stimulate the circulation.

Full immersion bathing is not advisable with some oils that can irritate the skin and/or mucous membranes. *See* A–Z of Plants and their Essential Oils, page 57.

Sitz baths

Sitz baths, or hip baths, are particularly beneficial in the treatment of menstrual disorders, thrush, cystitis, haemorrhoids and constipation. When treating haemorrhoids or vaginal thrush keep the water around body temperature, but otherwise the water should be quite hot. Tea-tree oil is particularly useful in the treatment of thrush.

NOTE

As with full immersion bathing, sitz bathing is not appropriate with some essential oils. *See* A–Z of Plants and their Essential Oils, page 57.

Compresses

Some problems respond well to treatment with compresses, made by soaking cloths or towels in either hot or ice-cold water – whichever is appropriate – and adding a few drops of essential oil. Cold compresses are useful for treating headaches, fever and pain from recent bruising or muscle strain. Hot compresses, applied to the relevant parts of the body, can alleviate menstrual cramping and muscle and joint pain and can be particularly soothing for chronic pain caused by arthritis and rheumatism. Hot compresses can also be used to treat boils.

To prepare a compress, fill a bowl with either hot or iced water, according to your needs. Soak a folded cloth in the water and wring it out. Add three or four drops of essential oil to the water in the bowl and swirl it round to disperse it thoroughly. Lay your cloth lightly back on the surface of the water, then wring out again and apply to the affected part for treatment.

If you are using a hot compress, place some polythene or clingfilm over the compress with another cloth on top. This will help to retain the heat.

If you are treating headache with a cold compress, make sure that the compress is well wrung out and will not drip. It is important that the essential oil is kept away from the eyes.

Mouthwashes

Some essential oils can be added to warm water and used as

mouthwashes or gargles to combat gum inflammation, bad breath, oral thrush and mouth ulcers. *See* A–Z of Plants and their Essential Oils, page 57. In order to avoid irritation of the mouth, the oil should be first diluted in a small amount of alcohol – vodka is generally recommended. Add two drops of essential oil to a teaspoon of vodka and mix into half a glass of warm water to prepare your mouthwash. Tea-tree oil is safe to add to warm water without alcohol, but this is the exception.

CAUTION
Mouthwashes should never be swallowed.

Skin care
There is a variety of ways in which appropriate essential oils can be used to benefit the skin. Facial massage with essential oils diluted in a base oil will stimulate the circulation, help to improve skin tone and impart the individual benefits of the essential oils to the skin. Dry, flaky and ageing skin will derive particular benefit from this treatment. Careful choice of an appropriate carrier oil will make the treatment even more effective (*see* Selecting and Using Base Oils, page 53).

Steam facials (*see* page 32) are an effective way of cleansing and treating skins prone to oiliness or acne.

Essential oils can also be added to unscented creams or lotions for application to the skin or, for the treatment of fungal infections and cold sores, diluted in a little alcohol (isopropyl alcohol is available from most chemists) before application to the affected area.

Neat application is inadvisable for most essential oils; but tea-tree oil and lavender oil are safe to use in this way. Tea-tree oil can be applied to spots. Lavender oil can be used on a variety of skin traumas: minor cuts, burns and scalds and insects bites and stings.

Lemon oil can be used to treat verrucas and warts but the surrounding skin should be protected with petroleum jelly.

Hair care

There are quite a few essential oils that can be used on the hair for a variety of reasons. Tea-tree oil, for example, will help in the treatment of dandruff. Rosemary will help to stimulate hair growth and condition the hair. Dilute in a carrier oil as for massage and rub well into the scalp. The oil can be left on the scalp for an hour or so. Wrap a towel around the head and leave, then wash as normal.

Vaporizers, diffusers, room sprays, burners

All the above may be used to add fragrance to a room with essential oils, letting the occupants benefit from smelling the odours that are given off. Certain oils can also be used as fumigating or disinfecting agents in this way, preventing the spread of disease. Others will make effective insect-repellents (*see* A–Z of Plants and Essential Oils).

There is quite a selection of devices to fragrance a room with essential oils, including electrically powered devices. Burners (a saucer-shaped dish above a candle in a holder) should always be used with extreme care. Use only the type of candle that is advised in the instructions or the whole dish might become overheated. Never place the oils neat in the burner dish: always float them in water.

Electric vaporizers can be bought in many large pharmacies. Make sure that they are suitable for use with essential oils.

Ring burners are also available: ring-shaped dishes that are fixed above a light bulb. Never allow any essential oil to drip onto the light bulb when it is hot.

One of the easiest and safest ways to scent a room with essential oils is to fill a bowl with boiling water, add some essential oils, and place it in the room with doors and windows closed for a while. Alternatively, place a bowl of water with essential oils added on top of a central heating radiator.

You can make your own room spray quite easily with a plant spray, some water and a few drops of the oils of your choice.

CAUTION

With one or two exceptions, the application of undiluted essential oil onto the skin is strictly inadvisable. Exceptions are lavender oil, which can be used as an antiseptic on cuts and scrapes, and tea-tree oil, which is useful in the treatment of spots and can be dabbed onto blemishes neat. Oil of lemon can be used on warts and verrucas but the surrounding skin should be well protected with petroleum jelly. If you notice any skin irritation after using any essential oils, discontinue treatment immediately. It is possible to become sensitized to some essential oils that you might have been using without any problems beforehand.

If you have sensitive skin, it is advisable to carry out a patch test with any essential oil that you would like to use. Dilute the oil in a base oil as you would for a massage blend and apply to a small area on the inside of your wrist. If you notice any redness or irritation within the next few hours, you should not use the oil.

Blending Essential Oils

If you make an appointment with a trained aroma-therapist, you will find that he or she will take time to ask you in some detail about your lifestyle and your medical history. Diet and exercise, sleep patterns, stress levels, mood, bowel habits, menstrual cycle if you are a woman – all have some relevance as they will help the therapist to draw up as complete a picture as possible of you, the patient, rather than 'it', the problem for which you are seeking help. All the information will help in the selection of oils that are likely to be the most beneficial to you as an individual and as a whole.

You will notice, as you read the A–Z of Plants and their Essential Oils, that several oils may share the same basic property; for example, quite a few have a relaxing effect, while others act as antidepressants. Within each group, there will be one or more that are particularly appropriate for individual cases, when other relevant factors are taken into consideration. Depression, for example, can manifest itself in different ways. A person who feels anxious, agitated and has trouble sleeping at night should be treated differently from one whose depression manifests itself in flatness of mood and lethargy.

When the aromatherapist selects which oils to use, he or she will also be considering which ones work in harmony with each other, both for fragrance and for effect. A successful, harmonious blend of oils that work well in combination with one another is known as a synergistic blend. As many as seven oils may be used in combination, but the art of blending is one that takes quite a lot of practice. When preparing blends at home, it is generally better to keep it simple at first and work with no more than four essential oils at a time. If you work with simple blends initially, you will gradually build up a repertoire of blends that you enjoy using. Write everything down as you go along – mistakes should be remembered so that you do not repeat them – and then, gradually, you will find that you are able to add to and alter your recipes. Successful blending takes a combination of time, patience, expertise and intuition. Remember, however, that it is not necessarily the case that complicated blends are more effective. Often, keeping it simple is better.

Mix your blends in small quantities. Once essential oils are mixed in base oils, they do not last as long. It is better to work with small quantities, making fresh blends each time, than to make up large amounts if you are not certain whether you are going to use a particular blend again in the immediate future. Blending small amounts also makes mistakes less costly.

In order to achieve a blend that is approximately a 2 per cent dilution, use six drops of essential oil to every tablespoon of base oil. For even smaller quantities, use two drops of essential oil to one teaspoon of base. Remember that some base oils have their own distinctive qualities; if you make a blend of essential oils in almond oil, for example, a light base oil that is virtually odourless and suitable for general use, it will not be the same if you use a different base the next time.

Blending guide

With time and practice, you will be able to build up your own 'menu' of favourite blends. The following may help you in your initial selection of essential oils in blends that you prepare. As a general rule, like blends well with like, so the spice oils can be blended with each other, the oils from the same plant family – for example *Labiateae* which includes basil, clary sage and hyssop – will work quite well together, the woody oils can be used in combination with each other, and so on. There are other broad guidelines that can be followed as well: citrus oils, for example, have an odour that is short-lived, but they blend well with the woody oils, whose fragrance is more lingering, so you can make blends that have a fragrance that changes in quality as time goes on. Perfumers consider that a good perfume should have a top note, a middle note and a base note. The top note is the shortest-lived, but probably makes the first impression. The base note is the longest-lived, the last lingering element of the fragrant blend. The middle note is the basis around which the fragrance is built – the substance of the perfume. Thus, in an aromatherapy blend, each oil will have its own distinctive qualities but, put together with others, will form part of a dynamic fragrance, changing its impressions on the individual all the time. Whilst this might sound a little complicated to the novice, it does serve to make the point that it is more than the instant first impression that counts when blending oils. If you are trying out a blend for the first time give it time. What is your first feeling about the blend? What comes through immediately after the first impression? What is it like after half an hour or an hour? How does it change?

Remember also that the therapeutic qualities of the oils that you choose should complement each other. Think of the outcome you are hoping to achieve.

Finally, if you are intending to give a massage to another person or are mixing a bath blend for the benefit of another individual, his or her likes and dislikes cannot be ignored. No matter how you might feel about the blend that you are making, it is the recipient who counts. In order for that person to get the maximum benefit from the oils, the blend should smell good to him or her.

Many books have been written on the subject of aromatherapy that give specific recipes for the treatment of certain problems, and these are very useful indeed, especially if you are looking for a 'springboard' to start you off practising aromatherapy at home. They will also give valuable advice on which oils, used therapeutically, are best to use in combination with one another.

The following is not a therapeutic guide. It is meant simply as a guide to some of the oils that are likely to work most successfully with one another in a blend. The proportions will vary according to individual taste.

Angelica
Blends well with citrus oils, clary sage, patchouli, vetiver.

Basil
Blends well with bergamot, citronella, chamomile, clary sage, geranium, lavender, lemongrass, lime, marjoram, peppermint, rose.

Bay
Blends well with citrus oils, clary sage, cypress, hyssop, lavender, myrtle, rosemary.

Benzoin
Blends well with black pepper, coriander, cardamom, cumin, cypress, frankincense, jasmine, juniper, myrrh, peppermint, petitgrain.

Bergamot
Blends well with basil, cardamom, chamomile, coriander, cypress, geranium, jasmine, juniper, lavender, melissa, mimosa, myrtle, neroli, petitgrain, sandalwood, ylang ylang.

Black pepper
Blends well with cedarwood, frankincense, juniper, lemon, marjoram, palmarosa, rosemary, sandalwood.

Cajeput
Blends well with cedarwood, eucalyptus, lavender, pine.

Cardamom
Blends well with bergamot, cedarwood, cumin, frankincense, neroli, orange, rose, sandalwood, ylang ylang.

Carrot seed
Blends well with cedarwood, citrus oils (particularly orange), geranium, mimosa.

Cedarwood
Blends well with benzoin, bergamot, black pepper, cajeput, cypress, frankincense, ginger, jasmine, juniper, lavender, myrrh, neroli, patchouli, pine, rose, rosemary, sandalwood, vetiver, ylang ylang.

Chamomile
Blends well with basil, bergamot, clary sage, jasmine, lavender, marjoram, rose, star anise.

Cinnamon leaf
Blends well with benzoin, eucalyptus, frankincense, lemon, mandarin, orange.

Citronella
Blends well with bergamot, cedarwood, geranium, lemon, mimosa, orange, pine.

Clary sage
Blends well with angelica, basil, bay, cardamom, cedarwood, coriander, frankincense, geranium, jasmine, lavender, lemon, myrtle, petigrain, rose, sandalwood, ylang ylang.

Coriander
Blends well with bergamot, carrot, citronella, clary sage, cypress, frankincense, ginger, jasmine, pine, sandalwood.

Cumin
Blends well with cardamom, coriander, lavender, rosemary, rosewood.

Cypress
Blends well with bay, benzoin, bergamot, cardamom, cedarwood, clary sage, frankincense, juniper, lavender, lemon, mandarin, marjoram, orange, sandalwood.

Dill
Blends with lemon, mandarin, neroli, orange, peppermint.

Eucalyptus
Blends well with cajeput, cedarwood, cypress, lavender, lemon, lemongrass, marjoram, peppermint, pine, rosemary, star anise, tea tree, thyme.

Fennel
Blends reasonably well with geranium, lavender, marjoram, rose, sandalwood, but many people prefer fennel used on its own because of its distinctive odour.

Frankincense
Blends well with basil, black pepper, cedarwood, cinnamon, citrus oils, geranium, ginger, myrrh, neroli, pine, sandalwood, vetiver.

Geranium
Blends well with basil, bergamot, hyssop, jasmine, juniper, lemon, lime, mandarin, marjoram, neroli, orange, patchouli, petitgrain, rose, sandalwood, tea tree.

Ginger
Blends well with cedarwood, coriander, frankincense, grapefruit, juniper, lemon, mandarin, myrtle, orange, palmarosa, patchouli, rose, rosewood, vetiver.

Grapefruit
Blends well with bergamot and other citrus oils, cardamom, cypress, geranium, ginger, lavender, neroli, palmarosa, rosemary.

Hyssop
Blends well with bay, clary sage, geranium, lavender, orange, rosemary.

Jasmine
Blends well with bergamot and other citrus oils, chamomile, clary sage, coriander, geranium, lavender, mimosa, myrtle, patchouli, peppermint, petitgrain, rose, sandalwood, vetiver, ylang ylang.

Juniper
Blends well with cedarwood, citrus oils, cypress, geranium, ginger, lavender, pine, rosemary, sandalwood, vetiver.

Lavender
Blends well with basil, bergamot, cardamom, clary sage, cumin, cedarwood, cypress, eucalyptus, geranium, grapefruit, hyssop, lemon, lemongrass, lime, marjoram, myrtle, neroli, orange, peppermint, petitgrain, rosemary, tea tree.

Lemon
Blends well with angelica, bay, benzoin, black pepper, citronella, citrus oils, eucalyptus, fennel, geranium, ginger, jasmine, juniper, lavender, neroli, peppermint, ylang ylang.

Lemongrass
Blends well with basil, coriander, eucalyptus, lavender, peppermint, rosemary, thyme, vetiver.

Lime
Blends well with basil, citronella, citrus oils, clary sage, lavender, neroli, nutmeg, rosemary.

Mandarin
Blends well with bergamot and other citrus oils, coriander, cinnamon, cumin, clary sage, geranium, juniper, lavender, nutmeg.

Marjoram
Blends well with basil, bergamot, cedarwood, chamomile, cypress, eucalyptus, geranium, lavender, melissa, orange, peppermint, rosemary, tea tree, thyme.

Melissa
Blends well with chamomile, citrus oils, geranium, jasmine, lavender, marjoram, rose, rosemary, thyme.

Mimosa
Blends well with citronella, citrus oils, coriander, jasmine, lavender, rose, sandalwood, ylang ylang.

Myrrh
Blends well with benzoin, cedarwood, cypress, frankincense, geranium, juniper, lavender, lemon, patchouli, peppermint, pine, sandalwood.

Myrtle
Blends well with bay, bergamot, clary sage, cardamom, ginger, hyssop, lavender, lime, rosemary.

Neroli
Blends well with all citrus oils, clary sage, jasmine, lavender, rosemary, rosewood.

Niaouli
Blends well with eucalyptus, lavender, rosemary, tea tree.

Nutmeg
Blends well with bay, cinnamon, clary sage, coriander, cumin, geranium, ginger, lime, mandarin, petitgrain.

Orange (sweet or bitter)
Blends well with black pepper, all citrus oils, cinnamon, clary sage, coriander, cumin, ginger, hyssop, jasmine, lavender, myrrh, neroli, nutmeg, petitgrain.

Palmarosa
Blends well with black pepper, cedarwood, geranium, jasmine, neroli, petitgrain, rose, rosewood, sandalwood.

Patchouli
Blends well with angelica, cedarwood, clary sage, geranium, neroli, nutmeg, orange, rose, rosewood, sandalwood, ylang ylang.

Peppermint
Blends well with basil, benzoin, eucalyptus, jasmine, lavender, lemon, lemongrass, marjoram, pine, rosemary.

Petitgrain
Blends well with benzoin, bergamot, clary sage, geranium, jasmine, lavender, orange, palmarosa, rosemary.

Pine
Blends well with cajeput, cedarwood, eucalyptus, juniper, lavender, lemon, marjoram, niaouli, peppermint, rosemary, tea tree.

Rose
Blends well with basil, benzoin, bergamot, chamomile, clary sage, geranium, jasmine, lavender, patchouli, sandalwood, star anise, ylang ylang.

Rosemary
Blends well with basil, black pepper, hyssop, lavender, lemongrass, orange, peppermint, petitgrain, pine, tea tree.

Rosewood
Blends well with all citrus oils, jasmine, lavender, neroli, patchouli, rose, sandalwood, ylang ylang.

Sandalwood
Blends well with bergamot, cedarwood, geranium, jasmine, lavender, mimosa, palmarosa, patchouli, rosewood, vetiver, ylang ylang.

Star anise

Blends well with chamomile, cinnamon, eucalyptus, lavender, orange, pine, rose, rosemary.

Tarragon

Blends well with basil, pine.

Tea tree

Blends well with black pepper, clary sage, coriander, cumin, eucalyptus, geranium, lavender, lemon, marjoram, nutmeg, pine, rosemary, thyme.

Thyme

Blends well with bergamot, eucalyptus, lavender, lemon, marjoram, melissa, pine, rosemary, tea tree.

Vetiver

Blends well with angelica, clary sage, jasmine, lavender, patchouli, rose, sandalwood, ylang ylang.

Ylang ylang

Blends well with bergamot, cedarwood, clary sage, jasmine, lemon, mimosa, patchouli, rose, sandalwood, vetiver.

Storage of Essential Oils and Blended Oils

Essential oils are best bought in small quantities. It may seem more economical to buy in larger quantities, but the more often a bottle is opened and the oil is exposed to the air, the more it will deteriorate. A larger bottle of oil may thus go 'off' before it is finished. Essential oils, kept properly, will last for quite some time; most will be usable for up to two years although a few, such as citrus oils, have a shorter life.

Store your blends in small coloured glass bottles, carefully labelled. The 'shelf life' of blends is shorter than that of essential oils. It will vary according to the oils that you have used, but two to three months is generally the norm.

Keep essential oils and blended oils in a cool, dark place; the refrigerator is ideal, but if you have very young children who have access to the fridge, a safer alternative is a locked cupboard in an unheated room. Alternatively, you can use a childproof lock on the fridge door. Some oils will become more viscous in colder conditions; remove these from the fridge when required and allow them to come back to room temperature and they will be ready for use as normal.

NOTE

If you do intend storing your essential oils in the fridge, it is advisable to keep them in a tightly sealed container. Once the oils have been opened, it is inevitable that small quantities will have dribbled onto the neck of the bottle and no matter how small the amount, the potent fragrance can spread to other foods in the fridge. Cheese with a hint of lavender is not to everyone's taste!

Purchase of essential oils

There are several places where you can buy a wide variety of essential oils. Many pharmacies now stock them, as well as herbalists and centres of complementary medicine. You can also order essential oils by post from some suppliers. Choose a source that provides information, or is willing to provide information, about the oils that it supplies – the keeping qualities of the oils, their uses, dilution advice, safety precautions, etc. A knowledgeable source is more likely to be a reliable source.

It is also advisable that you purchase oils that have a tamper-proof seal on the bottles. The more often an essential oil is exposed to the air, the more quickly it oxidizes. For this reason, you do not want to buy oils that might have been opened several times by curious customers taking a sniff!

As with food products, there is a growing demand for essential oils to be organically produced. Reliable stockists will have a range of organically produced oils in the selection they have to offer. Check that the oils that are claimed to be organic have a logo on the bottle from an organization such as the Soil Association (United Kingdom), which guarantees the reliability of source.

You can buy many products 'ready-made': bath oils, skin care products, etc. that claim to be aromatherapy treatments. Some (not all) of these products will *not* live up to their claims – check the ingredients carefully! Some 'aromatherapy' products will contain artificial, chemical substitutes for essential oils. These might smell similar, but they will not smell the same. Nor will they have the same effects. In addition to this, the base oil that has been used in the formulation of these products may be a mineral oil rather than a vegetable oil. Mineral oils are not suitable for aromatherapy as they are too heavy to penetrate the skin.

Finally, make sure that the essential oils you purchase are just that, essential, rather than a mixture of essential oil and base.

Selecting and Using Base Oils

There is quite a large variety of oils that you can use as base, or carrier, oils in aromatherapy. The oil you select will depend very much on personal preference and the purpose for which it is intended. The list below gives a summary of some of the many carrier oils that can be used. Individuals will always find their own favourites, whether for massage, as bath blends or for skin care.

Remember that base oils do not have an unlimited shelf life. Store in a cool dark place and do not keep for more than one year.

Almond oil
Almond oil has many advantages as a base oil and is probably a good one to keep as a stock item in your store. It is relatively inexpensive, bland and quite safe to use on most people. It is also, if cold-pressed, high in nutrients. Be cautious, however, about using almond oil on anyone with a known nut allergy, as a few unlucky sufferers will suffer a reaction to any nut oil on their skin. **Warning:** Always make sure that the subject is not allergic to nuts.

Apricot-kernel oil
Apricot kernel oil is particularly light, which makes it suitable for use on the skin of the face. It has no detectable smell. It is, however, quite expensive.

Avocado oil

Avocado oil is very rich in nutrients, in particular vitamin E, which makes it a good preservative, helping to keep essential oils that are blended with it fresh. Avocado oil is green in colour, and because of its heaviness people often choose to mix it with another base oil in a proportion of one to ten. It is good for the treatment of dry skin but is not suitable for those whose skin has a tendency to be oily.

Coconut oil

Coconut oil is particularly well suited to hair and scalp treatment. It imparts a lovely sheen to the hair. It is also very soothing and nourishing on dry skin.

Grapeseed oil

Grapeseed oil is light and virtually odourless. It can be used on its own as a base oil, or alternatively can be used as the main base to which a smaller amount (generally 10 per cent) of another richer base oil has been added.

Jojoba oil

Like coconut oil, jojoba oil is solid and waxy at room temperature, but it has the benefit of good skin penetration and is also anti-inflammatory, making it soothing on hot, irritated skin. It can be mixed with other base oils once heated, in one to ten proportions, and many people will go for this option because of the expense of undiluted jojoba.

Olive oil

Olive oil is suitable for use in the treatment of scalp conditions and dry skin. It does, however, have quite a distinctive colour and odour of its own, which not everyone will appreciate, and it is quite heavy. Some people will find it preferable to use olive oil in combination with another, lighter base oil.

Disregard the cheaper varieties of olive oil. Opt for cold-pressed virgin oil; the quality justifies the expense. As with all other oils, if you can find an organic option, it is an added bonus.

Peach-kernel oil
Very similar to apricot kernel oil in weight and appearance, peach kernel oil is also equally good for facial use.

Peanut (arachis) oil
Peanut oil is an oil that is very rich in minerals and vitamins. Some people with nut allergies suffer violent reactions to peanut oil, however. **Warning:** Always make sure that the subject is not allergic to nuts.

Sunflower oil
Sunflower oil contains vitamins A, B, D and E and is a cheaper option than some for use as a base oil. Be careful to look for cold-pressed sunflower oil, rather than picking up any old bottle of cooking oil from the supermarket. If it is organically produced, so much the better.

Wheatgerm oil
Wheatgerm oil is thick, rich and golden, and it is particularly rich in vitamin E – even more so then avocado oil. The vitamin E content helps to preserve the essential oils that are added to it. It is best used in dilution with another base oil,

in a proportion of one to ten, as it is heavy and viscous. **Warning:** Use with care on those who are sensitive to or allergic to wheat – test on a small patch of skin and wait for twenty-four hours to check for any possible adverse reaction.

Macerated oils
Macerated or infused oils are base oils to which herbs have been added. The herbs are left in the oil over a period of time to allow their properties to infuse the base oil thoroughly before being removed. These oils can also be used as bases or carriers for the addition of essential oils and have additional individual properties imparted by the herbs that have been added to them. Macerated oils include calendula oil (soothing), carrot oil (anti-inflammatory), and comfrey oil (healing).

Diluting essential oils for massage
Twenty drops essential oil = 1ml
1 tablespoon = 15ml
1 teaspoonful = 5ml

Dilution quantities of essential oil to base oil;
For a 1 per cent dilution: 3 drops per tablespoonful/1 drop per teaspoonful
For a 2 per cent dilution: 6 drops per tablespoonful/2 drops per teaspoonful
For a 3 per cent dilution: 9 drops per tablespoonful/3 drops per teaspoonful

A–Z of Plants and their Essential Oils

CAUTION

Some essential oils are unsuitable for use at home and some medical conditions contra-indicate the use of certain essential oils and/or massage itself. Read the information that follows with care. If you want to enjoy the benefits of aromatherapy in your own home, please do so safely, paying attention to the contra-indications that are given. Aromatherapy oils can be used by an untrained person quite safely to aid relaxation, relieve stress and treat minor aches and pains, but treatment of all other complaints should be left to the experts.

If you are currently undergoing medical treatment for any condition or using another complementary therapy such as homeopathy or herbal medicine, seek the advice of the relevant practitioner as well as that of an aromatherapist. This will ensure that any aromatherapy treatment is working with the other therapy most effectively. You will also be able to ensure that there are no contra-indications for massage or the use of certain essential oils in your particular circumstances.

Be sure that you only use oils that are safe to use and use them in the appropriate manner. If you have any doubts about using essential oils or massage, seek the advice of a qualified aromatherapist. If you have a serious or chronic medical problem, consult a doctor before considering treatment with aromatherapy. Do not make any attempt to self-diagnose. If you suffer from a skin disorder or have a very sensitive skin, seek qualified advice before considering the use of essential oils. Pregnant women should avoid the use of essential oils in massage unless they have absolute, authoritative information about which oils are safe for them to use and how they should be used.

ANGELICA – *Angelica archangelica/ Angelica officinalis*

The plant

Angelica belongs to the family *Apiaceae* (*Umbelliferae*), the plant family to which fennel, dill and parsley also belong. The plant is indigenous to Europe and is cultivated for commercial purposes in Germany, Belgium and Hungary. It is a tall biennial, growing to a height of around 6–7 feet (1.8–2 metres).

Angelica has been used in herbal medicine for hundreds of years. In China it is used for gynaecological problems and in Europe it is appreciated particularly for its value in the treatment of urinary and respiratory disorders.

The candied stalks of the plant are commonly used in cakes and confections, particularly in France, Italy and Spain.

The oil

Essential oil of angelica is produced by the steam distillation of the roots or of the seeds.

The oil is colourless or pale yellow and has a strong earthy, spicy fragrance. It is used for its fragrance in the production of perfumes, soaps and cosmetics. It is employed by the food and drinks industries as a flavouring ingredient.

Therapeutically, angelica oil can be used in a variety of

ways. It has a strengthening effect on the spirits and can also be used to treat nervous tension, anxiety and stress. It will give a boost to the flagging mind and body when fatigue has set in, particularly if this is stress-induced. Use in massage blends or bathing for this purpose.

Angelica can also benefit the digestive system, combating indigestion and flatulence and boosting a jaded appetite.

The effects of the oil on the circulatory system are primarily stimulating and detoxifying. Angelica also has a diuretic effect so can be used to combat fluid retention.

Angelica has expectorant properties so can be used to treat catarrhal coughs. It will also help to reduce the feverishness that is associated with coughs, colds and influenza.

Used in skin care, angelica oil is particularly good for treating dull, lifeless skin and will also benefit dermatitis and psoriasis, soothing associated irritation.

Suitable methods of use
Bathing, inhalation, massage, skin care, vaporizer/diffuser

Precautions
Warning: Avoid during pregnancy. Not suitable for use by diabetics. Avoid exposure to the sun – may be phototoxic. Otherwise, generally safe to use.

ANISEED – *Pimpinella anisum*
The plant
Aniseed is a member of the *Umbelliferae* plant family, which includes several other commonly used herbs such as angelica, dill and fennel. The plant is native to the warmer climes of Egypt and Greece, and is now also grown in several other

countries, including Spain and Mexico. The seeds of the plant have a pleasant liquorice taste and, as a result, aniseed is used in the confectionery industry and also as a flavouring for throat lozenges and cough preparations. Alcoholic beverages such as Pastis and Pernod are aniseed-flavoured and aniseed can be used as an ingredient in some recipes for home cooking.

Like fennel and dill, aniseed can have beneficial effects on the digestive system, combating flatulence, indigestion and colic. Aniseed also has a deodorizing effect on the breath so is used in breath-freshening preparations. Other properties of the plant have enabled it to be used since the times of the ancient Romans as an aphrodisiac, an antiseptic and a stimulant to the production of breast milk in nursing mothers. Aniseed also has a decongestant effect on the upper respiratory tract.

The oil

The essential oil is obtained from the seed by steam distillation. The oil is very pale yellow in colour and has a sweet and spicy smell. It is used extensively in the pharmaceutical and food and drinks industries.

Aniseed oil is used therapeutically in the treatment of respiratory and digestive problems but has a relatively high level of toxicity. Although the plant and seeds have culinary and medicinal uses, the essential oil is not recommended for domestic use.

Precautions

Can cause drowsiness and dizziness in large doses and is an irritant, causing skin problems such as dermatitis in some people. **Warning:** Not recommended for use in the home, unless on the advice of a trained therapist.

BASIL (SWEET) – *Omicum basilicum*
The plant
Basil belongs to the *Lamiaceae* (*Labiatae*) family of plants. The aromatic leaves and stems of the plant are a mainstay of many dishes in European cookery, adding a fresh, distinctively pungent taste to salads and sauces. Although basil originally comes from Africa, the plant is relatively easy to grow, flourishing in the area around the Mediterranean in particular. Even in the cooler temperatures of Great Britain it is a popular annual herb to grow, either in warm, sheltered gardens or in pots on the windowsill. There are several different varieties of the plant: French basil is the variety used in aromatherapy. Much of the basil that is grown for essential oil production comes from Egypt.

Whilst all cooks will be well aware of the versatility of basil as a cooking ingredient, not all of them will know of the beneficial properties of the plant when it is eaten. It is effective as an antispasmodic agent and thus its consumption is a particularly pleasant way to aid digestion. Basil has been used in herbal medicine for hundreds of years for the treatment of fever and stomach and digestive complaints.

The oil
The whole plant is used for extracting the essential oil of basil, which is obtained by steam distillation. The oil is either colourless or pale yellow and has a sweet, spicy herbal smell. Basil oil is used as a fragrance ingredient in the cosmetics industry and is also used extensively in food production.

Basil oil has many therapeutic effects. It is both soothing and uplifting when diluted in a base oil and used for massage;

it has the effect of relieving gloom and fatigue, generally lifting the spirits and promoting a sense of wellbeing. Massage with a blend containing basil oil can thus be a wonderful tonic for stress at the end of a hard working day and will also improve circulatory function. Bath oils containing essential oil of basil can make a soak in a warm tub all the more beneficial as inhalation and absorption of the oil both work their magic. Steam inhalation of the oil is a favoured treatment for many respiratory ailments, and basil is also known to be effective in soothing fever.

Basil oil will bring relief to insect bites and stings, applied in dilution, and also acts as an insect repellent.

Suitable methods of use
Bathing, inhalation, massage, vaporizer/diffuser.

Precautions
Avoid using neat. Dilute well to avoid skin irritation. Use with moderation. **Warning:** Pregnant women should avoid the use of basil oil.

BAY – *Laurus nobilis*
The tree
The plant family to which bay belongs is *Lauraceae*, the same family as camphor and cinnamon. The essential oil is extracted by steam distillation of the dried leaves and berries of the bay plant.

Bay, or sweet bay as it is also known, originally comes from the area around the Mediterranean, but is quite easily grown in sheltered, sunny positions in this country. The tree grows to as much as 60 feet high (18 metres) and is ever-green.

Bay leaves are a common addition to stews and casseroles, whether fresh or dried, and bay is one of the standard ingredients of a classic bouquet garni. The leaves are used whole and are removed from the dish once cooking is complete and their flavour has infused throughout.

In common with most of the herbs that are widely used in cooking, bay has beneficial effects on the digestive system. Bay can also help to combat flatulence, and chewing on a bay leaf will help to freshen the breath after a spicy meal.

History reveals that bay was widely used in ancient Rome and Greece. Apart from its benefits as a digestive aid, it was believed to offer protection from malign spiritual influences. The emperors of ancient Rome wore wreaths of laurel (another name for bay) in time of victory and it remains a symbol of victory, wealth and importance to this day.

The oil

The essential oil is extracted from bay by steam distillation of the dried leaves and twigs. The oil is yellow-green in colour and smells strongly medicinal. Bay oil is used for its fragrance by the cosmetics and perfume industries and is also used in the production of a variety of foods and drinks.

Bay oil can be used in massage, bathing and inhalation. It has an uplifting effect on the spirits, and medicinally it can help in the treatment of minor respiratory illnesses such as colds and influenza. It helps combat flatulence and indigestion and can stimulate a jaded appetite. Bay oil is an emmenagogue – it can induce menstruation – and can help when periods are scanty and irregular.

Suitable methods of use
Massage (well-diluted), hair care, inhalation, vaporizer/diffuser.

Precautions
Bay oil can be irritating to sensitive skins. Use in proper dilution and in moderation only. Those with particularly sensitive or allergy-prone skins should avoid the use of bay oil in massage at home. **Warning:** Bay should not be used during pregnancy.

BENZOIN – *Styrax benzoin*
The plant
Benzoin is the resin obtained from the tree known as *Styrax benzoin*, a relative of *Styrax japonicus*, or the snowbell tree, belonging to the family *Styraceae*. The tree is native to Borneo, Malaya and Java. It grows to heights of more than 50 feet (15 metres).

Benzoin in its crude form is a resin collected from the cut trunk of the tree. It is used in the East for its fragrance – primarily as an ingredient in incense – and also medicinally for infections of the urinary tract.

The oil
Benzoin, also known as gum bejamin, is an important ingredient in friar's balsam, or compound tincture of benzoin, which has been favoured for many years in the treatment of

chesty colds and bronchitis. The essential oil – or resinoid – is produced from the resin by solvent extraction and is very viscous. Some kinds are solid. It is orange-amber in colour. It is generally sold in solution. Benzoin can be used to benefit the respiratory system by steam inhalation, is an effective expectorant and has an anti-inflammatory action that soothes laryngitis. Additionally its antiseptic properties can help in the treatment of throat and respiratory infections. Its vanilla-like fragrance makes it enjoyable to use.

In massage, mixed with a base oil, benzoin is used as a stress-reliever, relaxant and mood enhancer. It is invaluable in soothing 'jangled' nerves and will warm body and mind, do much to relieve rheumatic and arthritic pain and stimulate a sluggish circulation.

Benzoin is generally kind to the skin and can be used as a cleanser and as a treatment for dry and chapped skin. It is also used extensively in the cosmetics industry as a fragrant addition to the ingredients in bath products, shampoos and perfumes.

Suitable methods of use
Bathing, inhalation, massage, skin care, vaporizer/diffuser.

Precautions
Friar's balsam, or compound tincture of benzoin as it is also called, can be irritating to very sensitive skins, but any irritation is likely to be caused by the other components in the tincture rather than the benzoin itself, which is unlikely to cause problems of this nature. However, there can be problems with sensitization to benzoin in a very small minority of people.

BERGAMOT – *Citrus bergamia*
The plant
Bergamot is an evergreen citrus fruit tree, a member of the family *Rutaceae*, which also includes citron, lemon, lime, orange and tangerine. The fruit is also known as sweet orange and is distinctively pear-shaped. It originates from Asia and can be grown only in warm climates because the plant is not tolerant of frost.

The oil
The oil has a sharp and pungent fruity fragrance and is easily extracted, from the rind of the fruit in particular, by squeezing the rind in the process known as expression. This is done mechanically nowadays, although originally it was done by hand.

Oil of bergamot has been used for its therapeutic properties for many centuries in Europe. In Italy in particular it has been used to treat fever and worms. It is also a fragrant and flavoursome addition to many food products – Earl Grey tea, for example – and an important component of many perfumes and scented products, in particular, classic eau de Cologne.

Bergamot oil is a powerful antiseptic. In appropriate dilution, it has prove its use in the treatment of many troublesome skin complaints, such as eczema, some of which can be reluctant to respond to other forms of treatment. Stress-related complaints such as headaches and irritability will often respond well to a massage with oil of bergamot in the blend. The effect of the oil is vitalizing and uplifting, soothing tension away without any sedative effect. The pleasant fragrance makes a lovely addition to a blend for a vaporizer.

Bergamot eases problem gastrointestinal spasm and flatulence and gentle abdominal massage can bring relief from constipation and colic. The oil is also detoxifying and is thought to help in the treatment of cellulite when used in massage. In addition to this, when used for bathing, bergamot oil can soothe inflammation and can help alleviate vaginal itching and the symptoms of cystitis. In inhalation or massage, it can be used in the treatment of respiratory infections such as sore throats and bronchitis. Bergamot can also be used in a mouthwash to deodorize bad breath and fight mouth and throat infections, or on the hair to control dandruff.

Suitable methods of use
Bathing, hair care, inhalation, massage, mouthwash, skin care, vaporizer/diffuser.

Precautions
Bergamot oil should not be used on the skin prior to exposure to the sun – it is phototoxic and can cause pigmentation. If possible, try to use bergapten-free oil which reliable suppliers of essential oils should stock.

BLACK PEPPER – *Piper nigrum*
The plant
Black pepper is the dried seed of the plant, a vine-like climber that belongs to the *Piperaceae* family and is grown for commercial purposes mainly in India and Indonesia. Its use as a spice goes back at least four thousand years and few cooks can do without it in their kitchen. Black pepper is highly

regarded in Chinese medicine, particularly for the treatment of digestive disorders.

The oil
Black-pepper oil is extracted by steam distillation of the crushed, dried peppercorns. The oil is usually colourless, sometimes with a greenish or light amber tinge, and has a warm, freshly spicy smell. Black-pepper oil is used extensively by the food and drinks industry and is also employed in the manufacture of some perfumed products.

Black pepper is a warming oil and can be particularly beneficial in the treatment of heavy colds, when the patient feels shivery, achy, listless and depressed. It is both stimulating and energizing. It can be used in massage or in a vaporizer. Used in massage, it will be of particular benefit to athletes and those with arthritic or rheumatic pain, poor circulation or chilblains, and it is comforting and warming in a footbath. Avoid using it in general bathing, as it can be irritating to the skin.

Suitable methods of use
Footbath, inhalation, massage.

Precautions
Use well diluted and in small amounts as it can be a skin irritant.

CAJEPUT – *Melaleuca cajeputi*
The plant
Cajeput, also known as white tea tree and related to tea tree,

belongs to the plant family *Myrtaceae* and grows in Australia, Indonesia, Malaysia and Southeast Asia. Cajeput is a very tall evergreen tree with whitish bark and white flowers. It is a commonly used plant in herbal medicine, in East and West alike, for the treatment of fever, respiratory and skin complaints.

The oil

The essential oil is obtained by the process of steam distillation from the leaves and twigs of the plant. It is pale greenish yellow in colour and smells fresh, herbal and medicinal. The oil is used extensively by the pharmaceutical industry and also in dentistry. It is an ingredient in cosmetics, detergents and cough and cold preparations.

Cajeput oil is quite an effective analgesic and can be used in the treatment of toothache when applied in a warm compress to the affected side of the face. Compresses can also be used to soothe the pain of strained muscles and bruises.

In skin care, cajeput can be used to treat insect bites if used in dilution. It can also help oily skin and acne.

Cajeput oil used in inhalation or massage can be particularly beneficial to the respiratory system. It is an expectorant and an antiseptic, and it will also be comfortingly warming to those who are suffering from colds and chills. The oil is one of the principal ingredients in Olbas oil, widely sold as a cold treatment.

In bathing, it also helps in the treatment of cystitis.

Suitable methods of use

Bathing (use very well diluted), compress, inhalation, massage, vaporizer/diffuser.

Precautions
Use well diluted and in moderation to avoid skin irritation.
Warning: It is recommended that cajeput is avoided during the first three months of pregnancy.

CARDAMOM – *Elettaria cardamomum*
The plant
Cardamom belongs to the family *Zingiberaceae* and originates in India. It is a striking, large-leafed plant, growing to about 10 feet (3 metres) in height. The seeds of the plant have been used in Indian cookery for hundreds of years and are equally popular in many of the kitchens of the Western world. The essential oil gives the spice its distinctive warming, invigorating qualities. Chewing the seeds can help to alleviate indigestion and heartburn and stimulate the digestive system into working more effectively. Much of the cardamom oil that is produced commercially comes from Guatemala.

The oil
Cardamom oil is extracted from the dried seeds of the plant by the process of steam distillation. It is either colourless or pale yellow and smells sweet, warm and spicy. It can be used in baths, massage or in vaporizers and its effect is warming, uplifting, invigorating to the spirits and imparting a sense of contentment to those who have been suffering from anxiety and stress. Cardamom oil is also believed to be an aphrodisiac and can be used in massage to stimulate a jaded sexual appetite.

Cardamom oil also benefits the digestive system, having a carminative (antiflatulent) and antispasmodic effect when mixed with a base oil and massaged gently over the abdomen. It can also be used in mouthwashes as it has antiseptic properties.

Suitable methods of use
Bathing, inhalation, massage, mouthwash, vaporizer/diffuser.

Precautions
Cardamom is generally non-toxic and non-irritant, but may cause skin irritation in some cases.

CARROT – *Daucus carota*
The plant
The carrot plant, a member of the *Umbelliferae* family, needs little introduction. A bright orange-red root vegetable with distinctive, feathery leaves, it is easy to grow, cheap to buy, a staple vegetable in the kitchen and rich in vitamins, particularly vitamins A and C. It is the seed of the wild carrot, a different variety of plant, from which the essential oil is extracted.

Carrot seeds are used in herbal medicine for kidney and bladder problems and also for some digestive disorders.

The oil
Carrot-seed oil is obtained by the process of steam distillation, after the seeds have been crushed. It is a golden oil with a warm, earthy smell. Carrot-seed oil has a variety of uses commercially as both a flavouring and perfuming ingredient in food and cosmetic products. It is used in aromatherapy primarily in skin care preparations, purifying and revitalizing tired and jaded complexions, tautening sagging skin and helping to heal pimples.

It can also be used in bathing and massage, its benefits being mainly to the skin but also relieving gout, arthritis and rheumatism. It can also help in the treatment of scanty periods.

Suitable methods of use
Bathing, massage, skin care, steam inhalation, vaporizer/diffuser

Precautions
None – carrot-seed oil is non-irritant and non-sensitizing.

CEDARWOOD – *Cedrus atlantica*
The tree
Cedar originates from the Atlas mountains and is grown in particular in Morocco, from where most of the essential oil for aromatherapy is imported. Cedar belongs to the family *Pinaceae*. The trees are large and imposing. Demand for cedarwood for building and furnishing has greatly depleted the ancient cedar forests of Lebanon, which is why the oil has to be sourced elsewhere. Another kind of cedarwood oil comes from the red cedar – *Juniperus virginiana* – which is grown in North America. Cedarwood itself is highly aromatic.

The oil
Cedarwood oil has a rich, honey colour and a warm, woody, sweet smell that appeals to both sexes. The oil is extracted from wood waste – sawdust, chips and shavings – by the process of steam distillation.

Cedarwood oil has been in use for many centuries. The ancient Egyptians used it in cosmetics and in the process of mummification. It is also used in incense. Nowadays, it is used commercially for its fragrance in a variety of household products and also in the manufacture of cosmetics and toiletries, in particular aftershaves. Aromatherapists use cedarwood oil for the treatment of respiratory ailments. It has antiseptic properties, and is effective against coughs, bronchitis and catarrh. Its use in skin and hair care is well recognized, and it can be very beneficial in the treatment of dandruff, eczema and acne. As an ingredient in a blend to perfume a room, cedarwood oil is warm and pleasant. The oil is particularly useful in treating stress and tension.

Suitable methods of use
Bathing, compresses, inhalation, massage, skin care, vaporizer/diffuser.

Precautions
Use in low concentration only as it can be irritating to the skin. **Warning:** Cedarwood oil must be avoided during pregnancy.

CHAMOMILE – *Anthemis nobilis/Matricaria chamomilla*
The plant
Both the above varieties of chamomile are used in aromatherapy. *Anthemis nobilis* is known as Roman chamomile, a low-growing herb with yellow, daisy-shaped heads that makes a soft and fragrant lawn when planted close

together. Roman chamomile is perennial, but German chamomile – *Matricaria chamomilla* – is an annual herb and grows wild in, amongst other places, both Germany and Great Britain. Chamomile belongs to the plant family *Asteraceae* (*Compositae*).

Chamomile has been well regarded in herbal medicine for many centuries. It is calming in effect and is useful in treating nervous tension and insomnia. The herb is also used for hair and skin care. Chamomile tea, made from an infusion of the flower heads, is a refreshing and soothing drink, good for the digestion and an aid to a restful night's sleep.

The oil
Chamomile oil is blue in colour and has many benefits, particularly in skin care. It is widely used in the cosmetics industry in soaps, creams and shampoos. Chamomile is known to enhance and brighten the colour of blonde hair.

In aromatherapy, the uses of chamomile oil are many. It is soothing and relaxing, and when used for bathing can alleviate stress and anxiety, soothe menstrual cramps and relieve tension headaches. It will also do much to relieve vaginal irritation and itching. In massage its effects are equally calming and can do much to relieve muscle and joint pain and to promote relaxation in those of a fretful or irritable disposition. Chamomile is invaluable in the treatment of skin complaints such as allergies, eczema and pruritis. Its action is anti-inflammatory and antiseptic. It has analgesic properties and is useful in the treatment of earache and migraine. In compresses, chamomile oil will help relieve painful breasts, especially in the early days of breastfeeding.

Suitable methods of use
Bathing, compresses, hair care, inhalation, massage, skin care vaporizer/diffuser.

Precautions
Chamomile is safe to use in most circumstances, nontoxic and nonirritant, although it can cause skin irritation in those who are particularly sensitive. **Warning:** Some therapists recommend that chamomile is avoided during the first three months of pregnancy.

CINNAMON LEAF – *Cinnamomum zeylanicum*
The tree
Like bay, cinnamon belongs to the family *Lauraceae*. The trees, native to Sri Lanka but now found in many other countries such as Brazil and Madagascar, are around 40 feet (12 metres) tall when they reach maturity. Cinnamon is a spice of age-old use. The trees are cultivated to form several stems at a time, and when the bark of the young twigs turns brown, the stems are cut. Cinnamon 'sticks', familiar to most cooks, are made from the inner and outer bark of these stems dried and rolled together. Cinnamon is a favoured ingredient in cookery both in the East and in the West. Its sweet, spicy taste makes it suitable for baking and puddings as well as for savoury dishes. Medicinally, cinnamon has a long history in Eastern medicine where it is used to treat fever and menstrual problems among other things.

The oil
There are two different oils extracted from the tree.

Cinnamon-leaf oil has some use in aromatherapy, but cinnamon-bark oil is a strong irritant, high in toxicity and should not be used. Cinnamon-leaf oil is extracted from the leaves and young twigs of the tree by steam distillation. Commercially, it is used in the food and drinks industry in some sweets and carbonated drinks, and in the pharmaceutical industry it is used in cough medications and dental preparations.

Aromatherapists can use cinnamon-leaf oil in massage to relieve rheumatism, and it can also be beneficial in the treatment of digestive disorders. It is a stimulant and is used to treat circulatory problems. It can also be of benefit to those who are suffering from nervous exhaustion.

Suitable methods of use
Massage (well diluted), vaporizer/diffuser.

Precautions
Cinnamon-leaf oil is a skin irritant. Use very well diluted and in moderation. **Warning:** Do not confuse cinnamon-leaf oil with cinnamon-bark oil, which is unsuitable for aromatherapy.

CITRONELLA – *Cymbopogon nardus*
The plant
Citronella is native to and cultivated in Sri Lanka, particularly in the south of the island. Another variety of citronella, which is grown in Java, Vietnam, South and Central America – *Cymbpogon winterianus* – is also used to produce oil. Citronella belongs to the plant family *Poaceae* (*Gramineae*)

Citronella is a perennial grass with aromatic leaves. The plant has a long history of use in the traditional herbal medicine of the countries in which it grows for the treatment of digestive problems and intestinal parasites and to combat fever. It is also used as an insect repellent.

The oil
Essential oil of citronella is produced by the process of steam distillation from the leaves – either fresh, partially dried or dried. The oil is yellow in colour and smells fresh and lemony.

Essential oil of citronella is used in the manufacture of some proprietary insect repellents. It is also used in household cleaning products and soaps.

Citronella is used primarily for skin care in aromatherapy. It is antiseptic and bactericidal and can be used to treat oily skin that is prone to spots. The oil is also useful as a deodorizer.

Citronella is a very effective insect repellent when well diluted in a carrier oil and applied to the skin. It can also be used in a vaporizer to deter insects from entering a room. It is an extremely useful oil to have in the home for this reason, especially in the summer months. Some gardeners use citronella to stop cats from digging around plants in the garden.

Used in a compress, citronella can help relieve headaches and migraine. The effect of the oil is uplifting and can help to cheer the spirits.

Suitable methods of use
Massage (dilute well), skin care, vaporizer/diffuser.

Precautions
Warning: Avoid during pregnancy (citronella is an emmenagogue). Can cause skin irritation, so always dilute well.

CLARY SAGE – *Salvia sclarea*
The plant
Clary sage belongs to the family *Lamiaceae* (*Labiatae*). It originally comes from Syria, but has been growing in Britain since the sixteenth century. It is an elegant plant with hairy leaves, growing to approximately 3 feet (0.9 metres) in height. It is grown in several countries now, and is cultivated on a commercial basis in Spain and France.

It has been used medicinally since the Middle Ages for many ailments, in particular eye disease – 'clary' may be derived from 'clear eye'.

Clary sage is safer to use than garden (common) sage and is therefore the plant of choice for aromatherapy. Common sage oil has a high level of toxicity and is unsuitable for therapeutic use.

The oil
Both leaves and flowers are used to obtain the essential oil of clary sage, the oil being extracted by the process of steam distillation. The oil has a distinctively herbal smell, light and quite sweet – almost flowery – with an edge that gives it a hint of bitterness. It is pale yellow in colour. Clary-sage oil is used by perfumers in France as a fixative for many perfumes and it is also used in the production of some foods and drinks.

Clary-sage oil can be used to treat a variety of problems. It has a sedating effect, calming tension and creating a feeling of greater wellbeing, while at the same time lifting the mood. It will be of use to anyone who feels weak and debilitated after illness, cheering flattened spirits and provoking feelings of optimism, and it is recommended for use in vaporizers or diffusers anywhere creative people are working as its effects are considered to be quite inspirational. Some people report that they have had particularly vivid dreams after using the oil. Used in large quantities, however, clary sage can cause drowsiness. Alcohol should be avoided if using the oil because the combination of the two can produce a strongly narcotic effect.

Clary sage is useful in the treatment of menstrual cramping – gentle abdominal massage or the application of warm compresses is recommended – and massage or bathing with clary sage can be of benefit to women who are feeling particularly low after childbirth, suffering from premenstrual tension or going through the menopause. Its antispasmodic properties can be helpful to both the digestive and the respiratory system, and when used for the treatment of stress it has the added advantage of being anti-hypertensive.

When used in inhalation, clary sage is beneficial to those suffering from colds or bronchitis; it is anti-inflammatory, antiseptic and helps in the healing process. The oil has astringent, toning, bactericidal and antiseptic properties that make it good for treating greasy skin.

Suitable methods of use
Bathing, compresses, inhalation, massage, skin care, vaporizer/diffuser.

Precautions
Warning: Avoid during pregnancy. Use in moderation. Avoid consuming alcohol if using clary sage. Avoid driving immediately after treatment. Not to be confused with common sage – *Salvia officinalis* – which is unsafe to use.

CLOVE – *Eugenia aromatica*
The tree
The clove tree is native to Indonesia but now grows in several countries. The tree is evergreen and of small to medium size. It belongs to the family *Myrtaceae*. Cloves, as we are familiar with them, are the flower buds of the tree, not yet open, which have been dried in wood smoke. Cloves have been a common flavouring ingredient in the cookery of several countries for many years and the deodorizing, antiseptic and anaesthetic properties of the essential oil have been appreciated by different cultures, in particular the Chinese, for centuries.

The oil
Oil of cloves is obtained by the process of water distillation from the buds of the tree. Essential oils are also obtained from the twigs and leaves of the tree, but these are more toxic than the bud oil and are to be avoided.

The powerful anaesthetic properties of clove oil ensure that it is a staple in the dentist's surgery. Dressings containing clove oil are very effective in cleansing and soothing holes in the teeth and aching empty tooth sockets. Some toothpastes also contain oil of cloves. For the treatment of toothache at home, put a drop of clove oil in a tablespoonful of warm water, soak some cotton wool in this, screw up a tiny ball of the cotton wool and apply this to the affected tooth; relief will be instantaneous, even if the taste is distinctly 'nippy'. Do not swallow. A safer alternative is to use tincture of cloves, which contains clove oil but is less concentrated and is available from most good pharmacies.

Clove oil can also be used by aromatherapists in massage for the treatment of certain fungal skin conditions and catarrh and bronchitis but is not advised for home use.

Precautions
Clove oil has a relatively high level of toxicity so it is recommended that you restrict its use at home to emergency dental analgesia. **Warning:** Clove oil is recommended to be used only by trained therapists.

CORIANDER – *Coriandrum sativum*
The plant
Coriander is believed to be indigenous to Asia and southern Europe but is now grown extensively throughout Europe and North America. The oil is produced in various countries, including Russia and Romania.

Coriander, a member of the plant family *Apiaceae* (*Umbelliferae*), is an annual herb, approximately 3 feet (0.9 metres) high with delicate, fragrant leaves, resembling those of parsley, and green, spherical, highly aromatic seeds produced in abundance. The leaves are used extensively in cookery and have a pleasantly fresh taste, almost orange-like. The seeds, either fresh or dried, are also popular in cooking and are an ingredient in many curry dishes.

Coriander has been used since ancient times. The tomb of the Egyptian Pharaoh Rameses II was found to contain coriander seeds. Coriander has been used in herbal medicine for the treatment of digestive complaints both in China and in Western countries.

The oil

Essential oil of coriander is obtained from the seeds, when ripe, by steam distillation. The oil is colourless or very pale yellow and has a fresh, sweet, spicy odour. Coriander oil is used in the pharmaceutical industry as a flavouring ingredient. It is also used in the manufacture of cosmetics, soaps and some perfumes. The food industry utilizes coriander oil as a flavouring agent.

Therapeutically, coriander is warming and stimulating on the nervous and circulatory systems. It is comforting and revitalizing and will help to boost confidence and combat debility when spirits are low. It is also beneficial in the treatment of muscular stiffness and aches and pains associated with rheumatism and arthritis. It has analgesic properties and will warm and soothe areas of pain and discomfort.

Coriander oil can be used to alleviate some of the symptoms of digestive problems, particularly when used in massage. It has antispasmodic properties and will relieve flatulence, colic and dyspepsia. It can help to stimulate a poor appetite, especially after illness. It can also help in the treatment of diarrhoea.

Coriander is useful in the treatment of post-illness weakness and 'blues'. It also has aphrodisiac properties and can stimulate a jaded sexual appetite when used in massage or in bathing.

The fragrance blends well with spice oils for use in a vaporizer.

Suitable methods of use
Bathing, compresses, inhalation, massage, vaporizer/diffuser.

Precautions
Coriander is nontoxic and non-sensitizing, and when used in dilution it will not irritate the skin. It can, however, have a stupefying effect if used in very large doses – moderation is therefore advised. **Warning:** Avoid using coriander during pregnancy.

CUMIN – *Cuminum cyminum*
The plant
Cumin is an annual herb, a member of the plant family *Apiaceae* (*Umbelliferae*) to which several other aromatic herbs such as parsley, coriander and dill also belong. Cumin originally comes from Egypt but has been cultivated in India and in Mediterranean countries for centuries. The fragrant, flavoursome seeds of the plant are a spice ingredient in many Indian dishes, and cumin has also been used medicinally in India, particularly as a digestive aid. Cumin is cultivated commercially in India, France and Spain.

The oil
Essential oil of cumin is obtained by the process of steam distillation from the ripe seeds of the plant. The oil is yellow and smells warmly spicy. Oil of cumin is used as an ingredient in some perfumes and also as a fragrance component in various cosmetics. It is used in the food and drinks industry as a flavouring agent.

Therapeutically, cumin can be used to treat digestive disorders and help in the elimination of toxins. Cumin oil is beneficial in the treatment of sluggish circulation and/or fluid retention, particularly when used in massage. It can also be used to good effect to assist the digestive process. It is carminative and antispasmodic so will combat flatulence and colic and soothe the discomfort of indigestion.

Cumin oil has a stimulating effect on the nervous system and can help in the treatment of nervous fatigue and weakness. It can also help to relieve headaches, particularly if these are stress-induced.

Suitable methods of use
Bathing, inhalation, massage, vaporizer/diffuser

Precautions
Warning: Phototoxic – do not allow treated skin to be exposed to sunlight within twelve hours of application.

In other respects, cumin is safe to use. It is non-sensitizing and non-irritant.

CYPRESS – *Cupressus sempervirens*
The tree
Cypress belongs to the *Cupressaceae* family of trees. This stately tree was believed to be sacred in ancient Greece and cypress branches were placed on the graves of the dead to facilitate their passage into the afterlife. Cypress trees originally came from the Eastern Mediterranean countries but can now be found throughout Europe. Cypress is often used as an ingredient in incense and is used in the cosmetics

industry widely, its sweet, fresh, invigorating smell appealing to both sexes.

The oil

Cypress oil is extracted from the young twigs and needles of the tree by the process of steam distillation. It is pale yellowish green and smells sweet, fresh and woody.

The oil is very refreshing when used in the bath or in massage, a great comfort for rheumatism, aching limbs and stress-induced fatigue at the end of a long, hard day. Cypress oil in the bath will also benefit those who are suffering from haemorrhoids, bladder irritation or the miseries of colds. Massage with cypress oil will help to relieve menorrhagia (excessive menstrual bleeding) and associated pelvic cramping. It will also help to stimulate the circulation. Its effects on the skin are primarily astringent and toning, and cypress has antiseptic properties. Used in facial massage, or in steam, it will benefit oily skin. It is soothing and deodorizing in a footbath and in steam inhalation will benefit catarrhal coughs and bronchitis.

Cypress oil makes a pleasant addition to a vaporizer in a room, adding freshness and energy to the atmosphere. Its effects on the spirits are stimulating, uplifting and energizing. It will also help to repel insects from the room.

Suitable methods of use

Bathing, compresses, inhalation, massage, skin care, vaporizer/diffuser/burner.

Precautions

None. Non-toxic non-sensitizing and non-irritant if used in dilution.

DILL – *Anethum graveolens*

The plant

Dill comes from the same plant family as fennel – the *Apiacea* (*Umbelliferae*) – and both the herb and the oil have certain properties in common. Dill is native to Mediterranean countries but is now grown all over the world for use as a culinary and medicinal herb and for the production of its oil. The oil is produced in several countries, including France, Germany, Spain and England. Dill is a tall annual or biennial plant. It has feathery leaves and yellow flowers and produces copious quantities of small aromatic seeds. Both the seeds and the flowers are used extensively in cookery. The gentle flavour, like that of aniseed, makes a pleasing companion to fish dishes in particular. Dill has been appreciated as a digestive aid for a very long time and it is one of the ingredients of gripe water which is used to relieve colic in children.

The oil

Two oils are distilled from dill: one from the plant, either fresh or dried, and another from the seed. Essential oil of dill is used extensively in the food and drinks industries as a flavouring, particularly in alcoholic beverages and pickles. Dill oil is also used in the manufacture of various cosmetics, toiletries and cleaning products as a perfuming ingredient and has some uses in the pharmaceutical industry in addition to this.

Dill oil is primarily used for the benefit of the digestive system in aromatherapy. It is carminative and antispasmodic so, when used in massage in particular, will relieve uncomfortable and distressing flatulence and colic. It also acts as a general aid to digestion.

Dill oil, like fennel oil, can be used to help promote lactation in nursing mothers. It can also be used to treat amenorrhoea (absence of mensturation).

Used in a vaporizer, dill will combine successfully with a variety of other essential oils to give a room a pleasant fragrance.

Suitable methods of use
Bathing, inhalation, massage, vaporizer/diffuser.

Precautions
Dill oil is nontoxic, non-sensitizing and generally nonirritant, although it may cause some irritation to those with very sensitive skins. **Warning:** Avoid use during pregnancy.

EUCALYPTUS – Eucalyptus globulus
The plant
Eucalyptus, a member of the family *Myrtaceae*, originally comes from Australia and Tasmania, but has been introduced to many other countries in the past two centuries, now being cultivated in Brazil, China, Spain, California and India among others. There are more than four hundred varieties of eucalyptus, but *Eucalyptus globulus*, or Tasmanian blue gum as it is also known, is the one from which the essential oil used in aromatherapy is extracted. Its history as a herb used in folk medicine stretches back several hundred years – the aboriginal people of Australia used it a great deal, particularly in the treatment of fever. The trees are highly aromatic, and it is wonderful to stand amongst them breathing in their aroma, especially after rain. Their presence in planting

schemes near buildings helps to deter insects. In some places the trees are planted as a preventative measure against malaria, and anywhere where eucalyptus trees grow will benefit from the fragrance and the healthy atmosphere that they give to the area.

Eucalyptus is widely used by the pharmaceutical and confectionary industries. It is a component in various cough medicines, throat sweets, ointments, sports liniments and toothpaste.

The oil

Eucalyptus oil is one of the most popular and commonly used essential oils. It is obtained from the leaves of the tree by the process of steam extraction. The uses of eucalyptus oil are many. Few people will respond negatively to its stimulating, clean aroma. Its effects are warming, invigorating and refreshing, and it has strong antiseptic, anaesthetic and healing properties. It can be used in steam inhalations, baths and massage, and it is particularly beneficial in the treatment of respiratory infections such as bronchitis, croup and tracheitis. When used in vaporizers and spray diffusers it not only deodorizes the atmosphere but also acts as a bactericidal fumigating agent. A vaporizer or a bowl of hot water, with a few drops of eucalyptus oil added, placed in the room of a person suffering from a stuffy nose or a troublesome cough, will do much to aid a restful night's sleep. A few drops of eucalyptus oil on a pillow will help to decongest a blocked nose and will be much appreciated by sufferers of sinusitis. During the day, a handkerchief to which eucalyptus oil has been applied can be used for inhalation purposes.

Used as an ingredient in massage oil, the warming effect

of eucalyptus is therapeutic for muscular pain and stiffness.

A couple of drops of eucalyptus oil in a sitz bath will help in the treatment of urinary tract infections. The bactericidal and antiseptic properties of the oil also make it suitable for treatment of skin lesions, but it must be used in dilution as it is very strong and can irritate the skin. It can be used to treat athlete's foot, insect bites parasitic conditions such as ring-worm and head lice, and it is soothing in the treatment of herpes and shingles.

Eucalyptus oil is an effective insect repellent, either used in a room spray or sprinkled on strips of ribbon hung from the ceiling (but keep these well away from light bulbs and heat sources).

Suitable methods of use
Bathing, compresses, inhalation, massage, vaporizer/diffuser.

Precautions
Eucalyptus oil is irritating to the skin. Always dilute well. Eucalyptus oil is potent and a little goes a long way. It does not have to be used in large quantities to have the desired effect: three drops will suffice for a bath. Use sparingly in blends to avoid the fragrance overpowering others. Some therapists recommend that eucalyptus oil is not used in early pregnancy. **Warning:** Eucalyptus oil is very toxic if taken internally.

FENNEL (SWEET) – *Foeniculum vulgare (var. dulce)*
The plant
Fennel is a tall, graceful member of the *Umbelliferae* family

and, although native to Mediterranean countries, grows freely throughout Europe. The plant is widely used in cookery, where its feathery leaves and celery-like stems impart a delicious flavour to many recipes. It tastes similar to aniseed. Fennel seed is an important ingredient in Indian cookery.

As with many of the herbs that are used in cookery, fennel has a beneficial, regulatory and balancing effect on the digestive system. It is antiflatulent, antispasmodic and gently laxative. Fennel tea is a popular digestive aid and anti-colic treatment. The herb is also thought to stimulate lactation in breastfeeding mothers.

The oil

Fennel oil is extracted by steam distillation from the seeds of the plant. It is very strong in odour, and in colour is clear with a slightly yellow tinge. It has bactericidal properties and is an ingredient in some toothpastes and mouthwashes, as it combats some of the bacteria that cause tooth decay.

Its antibacterial, laxative and carminative properties have made it popular with the pharmaceutical industry where it is used extensively. It is also an ingredient in some perfumed products.

Used in massage, particularly over the lower abdomen and back, fennel oil will soothe a nervous indigestion or irritated bowel. Flatulence and bloating can also be helped with gentle massage. Those who have problems with micturation often find that fennel helps to produce a steadier stream of urine. Its mild diuretic action can help with excessive fluid retention. Because of its strong odour, you may well find that fennel does not make a pleasing blend with other oils, but as its use tends to be more therapeutic than sensual, there is no need to blend fennel oil with other oils. Always dilute it well as it is strong and can irritate the skin – a $1\frac{1}{2}$ per cent dilution is quite sufficient.

Fennel can be used in vaporizers and because of its expectorant qualities is thought to help catarrhal coughs. Fennel has an effect similar to that of the hormone oestrogen – this is why it is used to stimulate lactation and increase milk production – and it is not suitable for use during pregnancy.

Suitable methods of use
Compresses, inhalation, massage, mouthwashes, vaporizer/diffuser.

Precautions
Sweet fennel can cause sensitization and should be well diluted before use. **Warning:** Sweet fennel can be narcotic if used in quantity. Do not use during pregnancy. Not to be used on people suffering from epilepsy. Bitter fennel (*Foeniculum vulgare var. amara*) should be avoided. It is stronger and more likely to cause sensitization.

FRANKINCENSE – *Boswellia carteri*
The tree
The tree from which frankincense resin is obtained grows in Somalia, China and Ethiopia. It is a member of the family *Burseraceae*. Frankincense was greatly valued in ancient times by the Chinese, the Romans, the Egyptians and the Arabs for its rich aroma and for its stimulant properties. It is to this day an important part of religious and ceremonial proceedings throughout the world and is used in the preparation of incense.

The oil

The oil is extracted from the gum resin by the process of steam distillation. It is an ingredient in a wide variety of commercially produced perfumed products. It is clear in colour, with a tinge of pale yellow. Its smell is woody, sweet and warm with a strong element of pine. It blends well with many other oils. It is both soothing and uplifting when used in a burner or vaporizer. Many people use it as an aid to meditation as it can help slow down breathing and aid concentration, and it is an invaluable weapon in the war against stress.

Frankincense makes a good addition to a steam inhalation – its anti-inflammatory properties are useful in the treatment of bronchitis and laryngitis, and it will also help troublesome coughs by soothing irritated mucous membranes and assisting expectoration.

Cosmetically, frankincense is particularly valuable. Its action is astringent, antiseptic and toning. It is popular in the treatment of ageing skin.

Frankincense is a particularly safe and comforting essential oil to use.

Suitable methods of use

Bathing, compresses, inhalation, massage, skin care, vaporizer/diffuser.

Precautions

None. Non-toxic and non-irritant if used in dilution.

Warning: Some therapists recommend that frankincense is avoided during early pregnancy.

GARLIC – *Allium sativum*
The plant

Garlic, a member of the plant family *Liliacea*, is grown widely throughout Europe and is renowned for its antiseptic properties. The plant has been used over many centuries in different countries as a protection against evil. Garlic also has antibacterial and anti-hypertensive properties and is greatly favoured as a flavouring ingredient in cookery worldwide, even if some people are intolerant of the effects that it has on the breath. There is no doubt that its consumption is beneficial to the health and if everybody ate it, the disadvantages of its smell on the breath – and in perspiration – would go unnoticed. Garlic capsules, which have all the advantages of large 'doses' of garlic but claim to be odour-free, are widely available in pharmacies and health food stores. Cooking with garlic and eating it, however gives much greater pleasure.

Because of its particular potency there is a little experiment you can perform using garlic that shows the effects of essential oils. Choose a day when you have not eaten garlic for some time. Peel and crush a garlic clove and rub it into the skin of your feet. Wait for an hour or so and then ask someone to smell your breath – remember, the essential oil would be much more concentrated in its effect than this!

The oil

Essential oil of garlic is a powerful antiseptic – possibly the most powerful among essential oils. It is unfortunate, therefore, that its overpowering smell makes its use virtually unbearable. It is just too strong and would never combine successfully with other oils. Aromatherapy is generally pleasant; the introduction of essential oil of garlic to an aromatherapist's repertoire would make both therapist and patient quite unpopular!

Precautions
Use of garlic oil renders all who touch it offensive to others.
Warning: Not suitable for use at home.

GERANIUM – *Pelargonium graveolens*
The plant
Pelargonium graveolens, a member of the family *Geraniaceae*, originally comes from South Africa. It is also known as rose geranium and is grown now in countries as diverse as France, Egypt, North Africa and Russia. It is an attractive plant to look at and, like all members of the plant family to which it belongs, a pleasure to see in flower. The leaves are highly aromatic and give off a distinctive smell when brushed against or rubbed between the fingers. Varieties of geranium have been used since ancient times in the herbal medicine of different countries.

The oil
Geranium oil has been an important asset to the perfume industry ever since it was first distilled in France in the early eighteenth century. The essential oil is extracted by steam distillation from the leaves and stems of the plant, which are harvested just before flowering begins, when the scent of the plant is strongest. The oil is green in colour and smells fresh and rosy.

The properties of geranium oil are varied, but in the main

it is an oil that is highly valued for its balancing, regulating qualities. It can be used in massage, bathing, or inhalation (either directly, in steam inhalation, or in a room vaporizer) and has the advantage of being generally nontoxic and nonirritant.

Geranium oil is often used in the treatment of menstrual disorders, especially premenstrual tension with associated fluid retention, and menopausal problems such as hot flushes. Its action is soothing and calming, and it works to alleviate anxiety and jumpiness, or restlessness, without having any unwanted sedative effect. It has analgesic and anti-inflammatory properties and, when used in the bath, will soothe the heat of acute cystitis and can also relieve some of the discomfort of chickenpox or the pain of shingles.

The anti-inflammatory properties of geranium oil also make it a favoured choice in the treatment of many skin conditions, such as eczema and acute dermatitis. It is also quite effective in the treatment of acne. Because of its balancing qualities, geranium oil can be used for the benefit of both dry and oily skins with no ill effects. In blends, geranium is one of the oils with a fragrance that blends well with many others, increasing its versatility.

Suitable methods of use
Bathing, compresses, hair care, inhalation, massage, skin care, vaporizer/diffuser.

Precautions
None. Geranium is generally perfectly safe to use in dilution on all but the most hypersensitive skins.

GINGER – *Zingiber officinale*
The plant

Ginger is native to Asia but is now grown widely throughout the tropics. The Caribbean countries, where the plant has been grown for some four hundred years, depended on ginger as an important part of the spice trade. The ginger plant is a perennial herb with a tuberous rhizome, and this is the part of the plant that is used. The ginger flower is white or yellow and very showy. The spice turmeric, familiar to all those who are acquainted with Indian cookery, comes from another rhizome, *Curcuma longa*, which belongs to the same plant family, *Zingiberaceae*. An essential oil is also obtained from turmeric but it is an irritant and not safe for home use.

Ginger has a long history of use both as a spice and as a herbal remedy, in particular for ailments of a digestive nature. Its effects are stimulative and carminative, so relieving flatulence. Crystallized stem ginger is used in the manufacture of sweets and preserves. Ginger-based remedies can be used as a remedy for both travel sickness and the morning sickness of early pregnancy.

The oil

Essential oil of ginger is obtained from the root, which has been previously dried and ground, by the process of steam distillation. It is pale yellow to amber in colour and has a spicy, sweet and pungent smell.

Ginger oil is used as a fragrance ingredient in some perfumes and is widely utilized in the food and drinks industry as a flavouring.

In aromatherapy, ginger can be used to help a variety of

problems. The oil is warming and toning and can boost flagging spirits and strengthen resolve. When used in massage, ginger is particularly beneficial in the treatment of musculoskeletal aches and pains that are more severe in cold, damp weather. It also helps to stimulate sluggish circulation and will work well on cold extremities. A footbath with ginger oil can be very soothing. Ginger oil can irritate the mucous membranes, however, and for this reason it is not recommended for use in full immersion baths.

Ginger oil, like the root of the plant, can be used to benefit the digestive system. It can be used to relieve nausea in the first three months of pregnancy and also travel-sickness. Inhalation from a handkerchief onto which one or two drops of ginger oil have been placed will bring relief. Ginger oil will stimulate a sluggish digestive system and will relieve associated flatulence. Use in massage blends or inhale for this purpose.

Ginger oil can also benefit the respiratory system, particularly if used in steam inhalation. It is an effective expectorant and so helps to clear the throat and nasal passages of excess mucus. It also does much to soothe an irritating cough and is thought to strengthen the body's immunity to the coughs and colds that winter brings. The oil will also help to reduce fever by encouraging sweating, which allows the body to cool down.

Ginger oil is an aphrodisiac.

Suitable methods of use
Compresses, footbaths (full immersion baths not recommended because of possible mucous membrane irritation), inhalation, massage, vaporizer/diffuser.

Precautions
Ginger is nontoxic and non-sensitizing. It should be used with care as it can irritate mucous membranes but is suitable for use on the skin in appropriate dilution.

GRAPEFRUIT – *Citrus paradisi*
The plant
Grapefruit is one of the citrus fruits that has a sharper, almost bitter taste. It is grown in the United States, Caribbean countries, Spain and also in Israel. It is larger than the orange or lemon and generally has a yellow skin. Pink grapefruit, less common but equally good, has a pink tinge to the skin and pink flesh. The taste of a grapefruit is such that it feels as if it is beneficial to the health, and it is. The sharp, fresh taste feels cleansing on the palate and wakes up the senses at the start of a day. Grapefruit is rich in vitamin C and is recommended as part of a detoxifying diet.

The oil
Essential oil of grapefruit is obtained from the skin and rind of the fruit by expression (machine pressing). The oil has a pleasant, fresh and sharp smell, much like the fruit, and is used by the cosmetic industry in many bath products, shampoos, soaps, etc.

The effects of grapefruit oil are primarily cooling, cleansing and detoxifying. A few drops of grapefruit oil in the bath act as a wonderful boost to flagging spirits. The bather will emerge feeling clean, fresh and new. In massage it can be used to help combat cellulite. Grapefruit is a valuable detoxifying agent and acts on the liver and kidneys to help the body to eliminate waste and toxins.

It will play a useful part in any detoxifying regime, and some people recommend it as an aid to the process of drug withdrawal.

Grapefruit oil also helps in the digestive process, and gentle abdominal massage will help to relieve a sluggish digestion or constipation.

Used in inhalation or in vaporizers, grapefruit oil combines well with many others in a harmonious blend.

In skin preparations, the actions of grapefruit oil are cleansing and astringent, making it ideal for the treatment of excessive oiliness. It has a similar effect in hair treatments.

Suitable methods of use
Bathing, compresses, inhalation, massage, hair care, skin care, vaporizer/diffuser.

Precautions
Warning: Mildly phototoxic so avoid exposure to the sun after treatment. Dilute well.

HYSSOP – *Hyssopus officinalis*
The plant
Hyssop is a member of the plant family *Lamiaceae* (*Labiatae*). It is indigenous to Mediterranean countries but now grows freely throughout Europe, in Russia and in the United States of America. It is cultivated for oil production in France, Italy, Spain, Hungary and the Balkan countries.

The plant is bushy and is a perennial. It grows to a height of approximately 5 feet (1.5 metres). It has small pointed leaves and flowers that vary in colour from pink, through violet to blue.

The herb has been used for many years in traditional herbal medicine, mainly for digestive ailments or problems of a respiratory nature, in particular coughs and bronchitis.

The oil

The essential oil of hyssop is obtained from the leaves and flowers of the plant by the process of steam distillation. The oil is colourless or pale greenish yellow and has a fragrance that is fresh and spicy. It is used for this fragrance in the production of soaps and other toiletries and also in the production of perfume. Hyssop oil is also employed in the manufacture of some food and drink products as a flavouring agent.

Therapeutically, hyssop has several possible applications, but it also has a certain amount of toxicity so should be used with care. Seek the advice of a trained therapist before using it at home. Hyssop oil is sedative in effect and can be used to treat anxiety, nervous tension and stress, either in bathing or in massage.

Hyssop is particularly beneficial in the treatment of respiratory ailments. It is antiseptic, antiviral and bactericidal and will help combat colds, influenza, bronchitis, asthma and sore throats. It also has expectorant properties that will help in the treatment of catarrh. It is antispasmodic so will soothe persistent irritating coughs.

Hyssop is an emmenagogue so can be used to treat amenorrhoea (absence of periods). Because of these properties it is unsuitable for use during pregnancy.

Hyssop can be used to regulate high or low blood pressure. Those who suffer from either problem should, however, seek qualified advice as it is important to find the cause in order to determine what treatment is appropriate.

In massage or in bathing, hyssop can also bring relief from flatulence and colic.

Hyssop can be used in skin care to soothe dermatitis and eczema.

Essential oil of hyssop should be used with care as it has a degree of toxicity.

Precautions
Warning: Not to be used during pregnancy. Has a degree of toxicity – use in strict moderation. Not to be used by epileptics. Not recommended for home use unless on the advice of a trained therapist.

JASMINE – *Jasminum officinale/ Jasminum grandiflorum*
The plant
Jasmine, a member of the plant family *Oleaceae*, originally comes from the northwest regions of India. It is an attractive climbing plant with delicate, pinkish-white flowers that exude a heady and delicious perfume. It is now cultivated for its oil in several countries, including Morocco, Egypt and France. Jasmine has been a mainstay of the perfume industry in France for many years now, in spite of the expense involved in the process of extracting its precious essential oil. The sensual qualities of jasmine have long been appreciated, as have its applications in skin care. It has also been used in the herbal medicine of East and West alike for the treatment of a variety of complaints.

The oil

Essential oil of jasmine is very expensive, simply because it is yielded in such small quantities. An astonishing amount of flowers is required to produce a small quantity of oil. The oil is extracted from the flowers of the plant, either by the process of enfleurage, a process still preferred by a very few perfume producers in spite of its labour intensiveness, or by solvent extraction. In spite of its expense, jasmine oil is highly esteemed in the perfume industry and is also an ingredient of many soaps, bath products, shampoos, etc. In addition, it is used to some extent by the food and drinks industry.

The oil is amber-brown in colour and quite viscous. Its odour is rich, sweet and strongly floral. Few people dislike the scent of jasmine, and it is widely appreciated for its powerful aphrodisiac qualities which affect both sexes. It is sometimes used as an ingredient of incense. Beware of cheap imitations!

Therapeutically, jasmine is valued for its antidepressant properties. Jasmine is useful in the treatment of emotional pain and stress-related depression. It induces a feeling of calm relaxation and can lift the spirits considerably. When used in massage, it will bring comfort to those who are sad or worn down by the burdens of life. It is beneficial during childbirth – diluted and massaged into the area of the lower back it will help to relieve pain and relax the mother-to-be. In sensual massage, jasmine will increase the pleasure of both partners, and it can be beneficial in the treatment of loss of libido or impotence, especially if this is stress-induced.

In skin care, jasmine is balancing and gentle. Its anti-inflammatory properties make it suitable for the treatment of irritated and inflamed skin in particular, but all skin types, dry and greasy alike, can benefit from jasmine.

Jasmine makes a delicious addition to a vaporizer in a room, giving it an air of cheerful calm, and it has also been recommended for helping to lift the spirits of new mothers who are suffering from fatigue and 'post-baby blues'. Jasmine combines successfully in many blends – the ease with which a harmonious blend can be created using jasmine oil adds to its versatility. The fragrance works particularly well in combination with citrus oils. The fragrance of jasmine oil is so powerful and long-lasting that, although it is costly, a little really does go a long way.

Suitable methods of use
Bathing, compresses, inhalation, massage, skin care, vaporizer/diffuser.

Precautions
Jasmine is generally nontoxic and nonirritant but can produce an allergic reaction in some extremely sensitive individuals.

JUNIPER – *Juniperus communis*
The tree
Juniper, an evergreen shrub/tree native to several countries in the Northern Hemisphere, belongs to the family *Cupressaceae*. The tree has needles that are bluish-green in colour and produces small, round black berries. The berries and needles of the juniper tree have a long history in traditional medicine and have been used to treat urinary disor-

ders such as cystitis, various respiratory disorders, gout and rheumatism. It was also believed in medieval times to have magical properties against the black forces of witchcraft. Extracts of juniper are used in veterinary medicine for the treatment of parasitic infections. It is an ingredient in many perfumed products.

The berries of the juniper tree can be used in cookery and are also used in the process of making gin, giving the drink its distinctive perfume and flavour. Juniper is cultivated for commercial production of the essential oil in Italy and the Balkan countries.

The oil

Juniper oil is produced from the berries and also from the needles and twigs by the process of steam distillation. The oil is pale yellow in colour, and has a pleasingly fresh and woody, warm, sweet fragrance. It is a traditional component of incense and has many uses in aromatherapy. Its diuretic and antiseptic properties make it useful in the treatment of bladder disorders and fluid retention. It also helps in the elimination of toxins, in particular uric acid, making it useful in the treatment of gout. In massage it will also help rheumatic problems and menstrual disorders and is warming and stimulating.

Juniper is beneficial in the treatment of stress and anxiety as it has a calming effect on the emotions and will help promote positive feelings.

Juniper oil can be used in skin care for the treatment of greasy, blackhead-prone skin and acne. Its action is astringent, cleansing, detoxifying and toning. Facial steaming will be particularly beneficial.

The fragrance of juniper combines well with many other oils, for example cedarwood, cypress, pine, lavender, geranium and citrus.

Suitable methods of use
Bathing, compresses, inhalation, massage, vaporizer/diffuser.

Precautions
Warning: To be avoided during pregnancy. May cause skin irritation in some individuals – dilute well.

LAVENDER – *Lavandula vera/Lavandula augustifolia/ Lavandula officinalis*
The plant
Lavender belongs to the plant family *Lamiaceae* (*Liberate*). It originally comes from the area around the Mediterranean but is now grown worldwide. It is commercially cultivated in France, Italy, Tasmania, Great Britain and many other countries. Lavender is an evergreen shrub with aromatic leaves and flowers, and it is a great favourite in herb and scented gardens. It has a long history of use – the ancient Romans used it in bathing and it has been used as a disinfectant, an antiseptic and a sedative. The dried flowers of the plant, sewn into a small pouches or bags, make delightful drawer fresheners. Lavender toilet water has been a popular product for many years.

The oil
Essential oil of lavender is obtained by steam distillation from the flowers of the plant. The oil is clear or faintly yel-

low and has a sweet floral odour that blends well with many other oils. Lavender is one of the most useful oils to have in the home as it is extremely safe and pleasant to use and has many functions.

The actions of lavender on the emotions are gently sedative and relaxing. It is beneficial to those whose low spirits are combined with a feeling of anxiety or vulnerability, imparting a feeling of calm while at the same time strengthening the spirits. It is a soothing addition to a massage blend and can help in the treatment of insomnia. Used in abdominal massage, lavender will help to ease flatulence and the discomfort of trapped wind in the digestive system.

The mild analgesic properties of lavender make it suitable for the treatment of headaches and muscular pain. One of the few essential oils that can be used neat, lavender also has antiseptic properties and can be dabbed directly onto stings and insect bites and will reduce the pain of minor burns, scalds and scrapes, combating infection at the same time. In addition to this, the oil promotes healing and will help to reduce scarring.

When used in bathing, lavender oil is beneficial in the treatment of genito-urinary infections such as thrush and cystitis. In steam inhalations, it can do much to ease spasmodic coughing and will help to fight throat infections and soothe laryngitis.

Skin conditions that can be treated with lavender oil include eczema, acne, psoriasis and athlete's foot. The oil has a deodorizing and antiseptic effect when used in a mouthwash.

Lavender oil is also an effective insect repellent.

Suitable methods of use
Bathing, compresses, hair care, inhalation, massage, skin care, vaporizer/diffuser.

Precautions
None. Lavender is extremely safe to use, even on babies and infants. Some aromatherapists recommend that it is avoided in early pregnancy if there is a history of miscarriage but otherwise it is very safe for pregnant women.

LEMON – *Citrus limon*
The tree
Lemon trees are evergreen, growing to a modest height of approximately 20 feet (6 metres). The tree is native to Asia but is now grown extensively in Europe, especially around the Mediterranean. The lemon tree belongs to the family *Rutaceae*. The fruits are bright yellow in colour when ripe, and both the flowers and fruit of the tree are highly fragrant. Lemons are rich in vitamins A, B and C and have for centuries been used as ingredients in cookery. Roman women in ancient times would take a drink made with lemon juice to relieve the nausea of morning sickness in the early months of pregnancy. The flavour of the fruit is sharp and the smell is sweet and fresh. Lemon juice used to be given to sailors as a treatment for or preventative measure against scurvy and has for many years been a favourite component of homemade cold 'cures'. Lemon is an ingredient in many commercially produced sweets and other confections and is used widely by the pharmaceutical industry, the perfume industry and the

cosmetics industry. Lemon is also used as a fragrance in many proprietary household cleaning agents.

The oil
Essential oil of lemon is extracted from the rind and skin of the fruit when ripe by expression. The oil is clear and has a light, fresh scent. It has a stimulating effect on the circulation and is beneficial to those who suffer from cold hands and feet and chilblains, either used in baths, footbaths or in massage blends. It has a cleansing and toning effect on the skin. The oil has antiseptic properties and is astringent, and it works well in the treatment of greasy, spot-prone skin and minor skin ailments such as boils and pimples.

In massage or inhalation, lemon oil's antiseptic properties will help combat respiratory infections such as colds, influenza, and bronchitis. In addition to this, it will also help strengthen the body's immune system.

Used in a vaporizer or spray, lemon oil is an effective insect repellent and will also help to disinfect the room of a sick person, at the same time refreshing the atmosphere and lifting the spirits.

Lemon oil is perfect for times when too many late nights and poor eating habits have given you a feeling of sluggishness or when a hard day's work or a long journey have left you feeling weary, sweaty and grubby. It is very much a 'fresh start' oil and gives an invaluable boost to the body and the morale.

Suitable methods of use
Bathing, compresses, inhalation, massage, skin care, vaporizer/diffuser.

Precautions
Lemon oil is phototoxic so should not be used prior to exposure to the sun. Apply in moderation and in low dilution as
occasionally sensitization can occur.

LEMONGRASS – *Cymbopogon citratus*
The plant
Lemongrass is a native plant of Asia, South Africa and parts
of South America. It belongs to the family *Poaceae*. It is a
majestic perennial grass, rapidly reaching heights of over 5
feet (1.5 metres) tall, and is highly aromatic. Of several
varieties that are cultivated, East Indian and West Indian
lemongrass are the two main kinds. Lemongrass has been
used as both a culinary and medicinal herb in India and Asia.
Medicinal use has been mainly for the treatment of fever
and infectious disease.

   The smell of lemongrass is like the smell of lemons but has a
harsher quality. It is very strong and is not to everyone's taste.
In cookery, too, it is not universally popular – it has been said
by some to taste like the smell of lemon-scented cleaning fluid!

The oil
Essential oil of lemongrass is extracted by steam distillation
from the cut grass. The oil is pale yellow in colour and has
an intense, lemony smell. It is used quite extensively in
industry in the manufacture of various food and drink products and also in the production of household cleaners and
bath and cosmetic products.

   Lemongrass oil has strong antiseptic, antifungal and
bactericidal qualities and can be used in the treatment

of athlete's foot, thrush, and feverish infections. Used in massage, its actions are warming and stimulating, and it will help to strengthen and tone weak, tired and aching muscles. It is thus useful for athletes and for those who are recovering, but still weak from periods of illness.

Lemongrass can also benefit the digestive system. Used in massage or in inhalation it can act as an appetite stimulant and soothe an irritated or inflamed colon. The antiseptic properties of the oil will help fight gastric infections.

Like lemon oil, lemongrass oil is beneficial to oily skin and can be added to a facial steam bath to help cleanse blocked pores.

The oil is an effective insect repellent and can also be used as a general-purpose deodorizer and air freshener, either in a spray or vaporizer.

Suitable methods of use
Inhalation, massage, skin care, vaporizer/diffuser.

Precautions
Lemongrass is non toxic but can irritate broken or sensitive skin. Use carefully and in low dilution. **Warning:** Some therapists recommend that essential oil of lemongrass is avoided in early pregnancy.

LIME – *Citrus aurantifolia*
The tree
Lime trees are quite small evergreens, bearing white flow-

ers and bright green fruit. The fruits are smaller than lemons and have a distinctive bitter taste. Limes grow in several countries and are grown commercially in Florida, Mexico, Italy and the West Indies. The tree is a member of the family *Rutaceae*.

Lime has been used quite extensively in herbal medicine for many years and shares most of the properties of lemon.

The oil
Essential oil of lime is produced by mechanical expression of the peel of the fruit. The oil is yellow/green with a strong, fresh citrus fragrance. It is used for its fragrance in the production of cosmetics, household cleaning products and perfumes. It is also used extensively by the food and drinks industries.

Therapeutically, essential oil of lime is more or less interchangeable with lemon. It is refreshing and cleansing and uplifting to the spirits. It has antiseptic properties and is astringent so can be used in the treatment of greasy and spotty skin. The bactericidal properties of the oil also make it suitable for treating skin infections such as boils.

Lime oil can also help in the treatment of respiratory complaints, such as colds and sore throats, catarrhal coughs and bronchitis.

The oil blends well with a variety of other essential oils and, used in a vaporizer or room spray, will also help to disinfect a room.

Suitable methods of use
Bathing, compresses, inhalation, massage, skin care, vaporizer/diffuser.

Precautions

Lime oil is phototoxic. After using lime oil on the skin, avoid exposure to sunlight for 24 hours. Generally non-sensitizing, but may cause sensitization in a few individuals.

MANDARIN – *Citrus nobilis/ Citrus reticulata*
The tree

Mandarin – or tangerine or satsuma, as it is now also known as, belongs to the family *Rutaceae*. The tree is indigenous to China, in particular the southern parts, but has been grown in Europe and the United States of America for almost two hundred years. There are quite a few varieties of the fruit, which are grown commercially in Mediterranean countries and also in Brazil, the Middle East and the USA. Both the flowers and the fruit of the tree are fragrant. The fruit of the tree is sweet and appeals to most tastes. The name mandarin has its origins in times of old, when the fruit was a traditional gift to mandarins, high ranking officials, in China.

The oil

Essential oil of mandarin is obtained by mechanical expression. It is orange/amber in colour and has a pleasantly sweet citrus smell. It is widely used in the manufacture of perfumes, soaps and cosmetics and also as a flavouring agent in the food and drinks industries.

Therapeutically, mandarin is a calming oil, soothing tension and nervous irritability. It is one of the safest oils to use in aromatherapy and is thus a suitable oil for using on children, who will enjoy the scent of a bath to which mandarin oil has been added. It can help in the treatment of hyperactivity and fretfulness in children.

Mandarin oil is also valued for the beneficial effects it has on the digestive system. Used in abdominal massage, it relieves colic, indigestion and constipation. It can be of great benefit to the elderly in this respect.

Mandarin oil is also a detoxifying agent and can help in the treatment of fluid retention.

In skin care, it is gently astringent and can benefit complexions that are prone to greasiness and/or acne.

Suitable methods of use
Bathing, compresses, inhalation, massage, skin care, vaporizer/diffuser.

Precautions
Mandarin oil is a very safe oil to use, but as there are doubts as to whether or not it is phototoxic, exposure to the sun is not recommended in the hours immediately after using the oil on the skin.

MARJORAM (SWEET) – *Origanum marjorama/ Marjorana hortensis*
The plant
Marjoram originally comes from around the Mediterranean. It is an aromatic, bushy plant, growing approximately 2 feet (0.6 metres) high, with small white flowers, tinged with bluish grey. It belongs to the family *Lamiaceae* (*Labiatae*) and is a perennial. It is often confused with pot marjoram, which is a much hardier plant. The herb has a long history of both

culinary and medicinal use. Its main medicinal use was for gastric complaints.

The oil

The oil of sweet marjoram is obtained from the dried flower heads and leaves of the plants by steam distillation. It is yellow-gold in colour and has a warm, spicy smell. It is used in the food and drinks industries and in the manufacture of scented bath products, cosmetics, perfumes and household cleaning products.

Marjoram oil has sedative properties and can help in the treatment of insomnia and tension. For those who are distraught with grief, 'wound up' with stress or highly emotional, marjoram can work to restore calmness of mind.

The sedative effects of marjoram mean that it is also an anaphrodisiac, that is, it reduces sexual urges.

Used in massage oil, in compresses or in baths, marjoram is valuable in the treatment of arthritis, muscular pain and swelling. It is analgesic and warming. For this reason, it can relieve dysmenorrhoea (painful menstruation). Marjoram oil is also an emmenagogue so is sometimes used in the treatment of amenorrhoea (absence of menstruation) and premenstrual tension.

In massage or in steam inhalation, marjoram oil can soothe the pain of sinusitis and headaches, including migraine.

The actions of marjoram oil on the digestive system are carminative (antiflatulence) and antispasmodic.

In massage or in bathing, marjoram oil can soothe areas of bruising and relieve the pain of chilblains.

Suitable methods of use

Bathing, compresses, inhalation, massage, vaporizer/diffuser.

Precautions

Although its sedative effects can be quite marked, marjoram is generally safe to use in appropriate dilution. **Warning:** Because of its properties as an emmenagogue, marjoram should not be used during pregnancy.

MELISSA (TRUE) – *Melissa officinalis*
The plant

Melissa officinalis, also known as lemon balm, is a fragrant-smelling herb with bright green leaves and tiny white flowers. It belongs to the family *Lamiaceae* (*Labiatae*), originally comes from the Mediterranean but is now grown extensively throughout Europe and is cultivated commercially in France, Spain and Russia. It is growing in popularity as a garden plant and culinary herb and also has a very long history of use in herbal medicine, being used to treat depression and nervous, respiratory, menstrual and digestive disorders.

The oil

The essential oil is obtained from the leaves and flowers of the plant by the process of steam distillation. The plant yields very small quantities of essential oil and therefore the oil is rather costly to produce and to buy. True melissa oil will be very expensive indeed, and it is often the case that melissa is combined with lemongrass before it is sold. The consumer must be on his or her guard, both for adulterated oil such as this and also for synthetic products.

Melissa is used for its fragrance in the manufacture of perfumed products and is also a flavouring ingredient in a variety of commercially produced food and drinks.

Therapeutically, melissa is uplifting and soothing and is

useful in times of grief, trauma and associated depression. It can also be used to treat insomnia and headaches, in particular migraine.

Melissa oil can also benefit the digestive and respiratory systems. It is antispasmodic and will help in the treatment of colic and feelings of nausea. Irritating coughs and bronchitis should respond well to steam inhalation with melissa.

Suitable methods of use
Bathing, inhalation, massage, vaporizer/diffuser

Precautions
Melissa is nontoxic, but can cause sensitization and/or skin irritation in a minority of individuals. Use well diluted.

MIMOSA – *Acacia dealbata*
The tree
Mimosa, a member of the family *Mimosaceae*, is native to Australia where it is also known as Sydney black wattle. It is a relatively small tree that has sweet-smelling yellow flowers. It has now become naturalized in several other countries in Africa and Europe. The bark of the mimosa tree is used in the tanning industry. It is also valued in herbal medicine for the treatment of diarrhoea amongst other things.

The oil
The essential oil is obtained by solvent extraction, which produces a solid concrete and a thick liquid absolute. The absolute is yellow-gold in colour and viscous. It has a woody,

warm and floral scent. The properties that make mimosa beneficial for therapeutic massage are principally its sooth-ing qualities – it has an uplifting effect on the spirits and can help those who are suffering from fear, anxiety and stress. It is mildly astringent and anti-inflammatory, and it is a valu-able component in a skin-care regime, benefiting oily and sensitive skin in particular, but it is very expensive.

Mimosa is used extensively by the perfume and cosmetics industries.

Suitable methods of use
Bathing, massage, skin care, vaporizer/diffuser.

Precautions
None. Mimosa is non-toxic, non-sensitizing and non-irri-tant.

MYRRH – *Commiphora myrrha*
The plant
Myrrh is a small shrub-like tree that grows to a height of 20–30 feet (6–9 metres). Belonging to the family *Burseraceae*, it is indigenous to Arabia, in particular Yemen, and to parts of northeast Africa, including Somalia and Ethiopia. The tree has white flowers and aromatic leaves. The trunk exudes a yellow liquid resin that hardens into solid reddish-coloured droplets. Resin collectors make incisions in the trunk of the tree to encourage it to produce larger quantities.

Myrrh, one of the gifts that the three wise men brought from the East for the Christ child, has been used since ancient times in religious ceremonies and is an ingredient of incense.

The ancient Egyptians used myrrh for embalming their dead. In herbal medicine, myrrh has a history of use as a tonic, with astringent and healing properties. It was also used as an expectorant and as a treatment for various gastric and oral problems and skin problems.

The oil

Myrrh oil is obtained by steam distillation from the resin that is exuded from the tree. It is golden to amber in colour and has a sweetish spicy, medicinal smell. It has strong antiseptic and healing properties. When used in the treatment of respiratory disorders, either in massage or in steam inhalation, its anti-inflammatory, anticatarrhal and expectorant properties can benefit coughs, bronchitis and sore throats. It can also be used in mouthwashes and gargles to treat gingivitis, mouth ulcers and oral thrush.

The effects of myrrh oil on the digestive system are stimulating. Used in massage, myrrh can help ease flatulence and stimulate appetite. It can also be used in the treatment of diarrhoea.

In skin care, either in the bath or in lotions or compresses, myrrh can be used as an antiseptic and anti-inflammatory agent. It works well on cracked and inflamed skin and can be used as a treatment for fungal infections such as athlete's foot and ringworm. In baths it can be used for the treatment of leucorrhoea and vaginal thrush. Myrrh is also thought to benefit ageing skin.

Myrrh oil is warming and relaxing and can be useful in the treatment of stress and depression. It is also used as an aid to meditation.

Myrrh oil is used in the cosmetics industry as an ingredient in soaps, cosmetics and perfumes. The pharmaceutical industry uses it in the production of oral preparations such as toothpastes and mouthwashes. It is also used in dentistry.

Suitable methods of use
Bathing, inhalation, massage, mouthwashes, skin care, vaporizer/diffuser.

Precautions
Myrrh oil is nonirritant and nontoxic when used externally. **Warning:** Do not swallow mouthwash. Not to be used in pregnancy.

MYRTLE – *Myrtus communis*
The plant
Myrtle is a large bush, growing to a height of as much as 15 feet (4.5 metres), which is native to North Africa but now growing throughout the Mediterranean area. It is an ever-green plant with shiny leaves and bright white blossom. Both leaves and flowers are fragrant. In ancient times, myrtle was sacred to the goddess Aphrodite, and it is still worn as a symbol of purity by some brides to this day. Like tea tree and eucalyptus, myrtle is a member of the plant family *Myrtaceae*. Myrtle oil is produced in several countries, including France, Morocco, Italy and Tunisia.

In traditional herbal medicine, myrtle has been used for respiratory and digestive disorders and also in skin care.

The oil
The essential oil of myrtle is obtained by steam distillation from the twigs and leaves of the plant. It is pale yellow to

orange in colour and has a clean fresh smell. The oil is used in the perfume industry, particularly in the production of eau de Cologne. It is also used as a flavouring ingredient in some commercially produced savoury foods.

Therapeutically, myrtle oil is used in aromatherapy for the treatment of respiratory complaints and also in skin care. Myrtle can be used to combat problem catarrh and coughing associated with this. It is also a useful treatment for sinusitis. It is bactericidal and an effective expectorant. Use in steam inhalation for best effect. The oil will also boost the immune system against colds and influenza.

In skin care, myrtle is useful for its astringent and bactericidal properties and can be used in skin preparations to treat oily skin and acne.

Myrtle has a clarifying and uplifting effect on the spirits. It can help those who are feeling low and distracted by worry.

Suitable methods of use
Bathing, inhalation, massage, skin care, vaporizer/diffuser.

Precautions
None. Myrtle is nontoxic, non-sensitizing and nonirritant.

NEROLI – *Citrus aurantium var. amara* (*see also* ORANGE (BITTER) and PETITGRAIN)
The tree
Neroli, also known as orange blossom, is derived from the flowers of the bitter orange tree, also known as the Seville orange. The tree, a member of the family *Rutaceae*, is indigenous to the Far East but is now grown extensively in

Mediterranean countries. The tree is a small evergreen, growing to heights of little more than 30 feet (9 metres). It has fragrant white flowers and dark orange-coloured fruits. The flowers were used traditionally in bridal bouquets as their perfume would calm the nervous bride before her wedding night. Dried flowers of bitter orange are also used in herbal medicine, taken in infusion as a tonic and blood-cleanser. Orange-flower water has been for a long time a popular aid in skin care for cleansing and toning.

Bitter oranges are used extensively in the food and drinks industry.

The oil

Neroli is named after an Italian princess who lived in the sixteenth century and is said to have used the oil as a perfume. Neroli is an ingredient in the classic eau de Cologne and many other perfumes. The oil is obtained from the flowers by steam distillation and is pale yellow in colour with a fragrance that is fresh and floral with a hint of sharpness underneath. Although neroli is quite an expensive essential oil to buy, it is much favoured by therapists as it has many therapeutic properties and is a very safe oil to use. It is both sedative and antidepressant and is very valuable in the treatment of feelings of anxiety and nervous tension as it is calming and soothing. It is often used in the treatment of premenstrual tension, helping to balance the mood swings that are often associated with this condition. In bathing, inhalation or massage it will benefit those who have trouble sleeping, especially if the insomnia is related to distress or anxiety. It will also soothe nervous palpitations.

Neroli benefits the digestive system with its antispasmodic

properties. Used in massage, in particular abdominal massage, it can help to ease colic, flatulence and stress-related colitis and diarrhoea.

In skin care, neroli is particularly beneficial to mature skins, having a rejuvenating effect. It is quite safe to use in dilution on sensitive skin and is helpful in preventing scars and stretchmarks.

Neroli combines especially well in a blend with jasmine and rose – very expensive, but quite wonderful.

Suitable methods of use
Bathing, inhalation, massage, skin care, vaporizer/diffuser.

Precautions
None. Neroli is nontoxic, non-sensitizing and nonirritant. It is one of the safest oils to use in home aromatherapy.

NIAOULI – *Melaleuca viridiflora*
The tree
Niaouli is a member of the family *Myrtaceae* and is an evergreen tree with yellow flowers and very aromatic leaves. It is indigenous to Australia and some of the islands of the Pacific. Most of the oil produced commercially comes from Australia. Niaouli is still used in herbal medicine in some of the places where it grows for the treatment of respiratory disease and for antisepsis amongst other things. Niaouli is related to cajeput and tea tree and shares some of their properties.

The oil
Essential oil of niaouli is obtained from the leaves of the

tree and also from young twigs by the process of steam distillation. The oil is generally colourless, or can be faintly greenish-yellow. It smells warm, sweet and quite like camphor. The essential oil is used quite extensively in the pharmaceutical industry, in particular for the manufacture of antiseptic throat and mouth preparations such as cough sweets and mouthwashes.

Niaouli has a variety of uses in aromatherapy. It can be used to treat respiratory tract infections such as sinusitis and bronchitis, especially when used in steam inhalation, and it is particularly beneficial in cases where mucus and catarrh are a problem.

Niaouli can also be used to treat various skin complaints. It is astringent and thus appropriate for the treatment of oily skin that is prone to acne. Insect bites and minor cuts, abrasions and burns can also be treated with preparations containing this essential oil, which has both antiseptic and analgesic properties.

When used in bathing or in massage (particularly massage), niaouli will bring some relief to the discomfort of rheumatism and general musculo-skeletal aches and pains. It also helps to stimulate the circulation.

Niaouli has a generally stimulating effect on the mind, clearing confusion and helping with focus and concentration.

Suitable methods of use
Bathing, inhalation, massage, skin care, vaporizer/diffuser

Precautions
Nonirritant and nontoxic. Non-sensitizing.
Warning: Avoid during the early months of pregnancy.

NUTMEG – *Myristica fragrans*
The tree

Nutmeg is native to the Middle East and the West Indies, and is cultivated in the West Indies, Indonesia and Sri Lanka. The tree is about 25 feet (7.6 metres) high and has aromatic leaves. The spice mace is obtained from the covering of the seed shell. Nutmeg is the kernel, which has been dried over heat in its shell. The spice has been used in cookery for many years. Nutmeg has been used in herbal medicine for hundreds of years, mostly for the treatment of digestive complaints, such as flatulence, indigestion and diarrhoea, and also for kidney disorders.

The oil

Essential oil of nutmeg is obtained from the dried seeds by steam distillation. The oil is white or pale yellow in colour. It has stimulant and analgesic properties and is warming in its effect when used in massage. It is beneficial in the treatment of muscular aches and pains, rheumatism and arthritis. It can also help in the treatment of digestive problems, such as flatulence, indigestion and nausea, and can stimulate a jaded appetite. Its effects are calming and strengthening and can benefit those who are chronically tired, depressed and lacking in energy. Nutmeg oil is not recommended for home use as it can, when used in high dose, cause hallucinations and hypnosis. It is unsuitable for bathing as it is a skin irritant.

Precautions

Warning: Use only under the supervision of a trained aromatherapist. Not suitable for bathing. Avoid during pregnancy.

ORANGE (BITTER) – *Citrus aurantium var. amara* (*see also* NEROLI and PETITGRAIN)

The tree

The bitter – or Seville – orange tree is also the source of the flowers that are used to obtain neroli oil (*see* page 120). It is an evergreen, a member of the family *Rutaceae* and although native to the Far East has been growing in the countries around the Mediterranean for many years. The tree grows to a height of approximately 30 feet (9 metres). The branches have very sharp spines. The flowers of the bitter orange tree are highly fragrant. The fruit is too bitter to be enjoyable when consumed raw but is used extensively in the food and drinks industries as a flavouring ingredient and in the making of marmalade.

In herbal medicine, bitter orange peel, dried, is used in moderate quantities in treating flatulence and dyspepsia.

The oil

The oil of the bitter orange is obtained by mechanical expression of the fruit peel. It is pale orange in colour and has a fresh, rich citrus scent that is not long-lasting. In common with other citrus oils, bitter orange has a relatively poor keeping quality. Like neroli, bitter orange is soothing to the nervous system and will benefit stress- and anxiety-related problems when used in massage or in bathing. It is useful in skin care for the treatment of oily and lacklustre complexions. It is astringent, anti-inflammatory and bactericidal.

Bitter orange oil, used in massage, will have a carminative (antiflatulent) effect on the digestive system and can also help to stimulate the digestion, encourage peristalsis and ease constipation. It is also useful in the treatment of water reten-tion and has a generally detoxifying effect.

In steam inhalation or in vaporizers, bitter orange oil has a relaxing effect while at the same time encouraging a more optimistic and cheerful outlook.

Suitable methods of use
Bathing, compresses, inhalation, massage, skin care, vapor-izer/diffuser.

Precautions
Warning: Phototoxic – Avoid exposure to sunlight for twelve hours following application. Otherwise generally non sensi-tizing and nonirritating although a very small number of people experience some skin irritation after using the oil.

ORANGE (SWEET) – *Citrus sinensis*
The tree
A member of the family *Rutaceae*, the sweet orange is a smaller tree than the bitter orange tree and, unlike the bitter orange tree, has spineless branches. The sweet orange is native to the Far East but has been grown in Mediterranean countries, especially in Spain. It is also widely grown in Portugal and in Brazil and the United States, where it is cultivated for oil production. The flowers of the sweet or-ange tree are fragrant, but their scent is not as strong as bit-ter orange blossom. Sweet oranges are almost universally popular for their pleasant taste and are high in vitamin C. Many varieties are cultivated for consumption and for uti-lization in the production of a variety of foods and drinks.

The oil

Sweet orange oil is obtained by mechanical expression of the peel of the fruit. It is light orange in colour and has a fresh, fruity smell that is sweeter in tone than that of the bitter orange. Sweet orange oil is a very safe oil to use in the home for aromatherapy and can be used on children, who generally enjoy the pleasant fragrance. Like other citrus oils, however, it has a relatively short life. Its therapeutic uses are many.

Sweet orange oil is very useful in skin care and is suitable for adding to the bath or for use in massage. It is gently astringent, conditioning and toning, and works well on all but the driest of skins, renewing a dull complexion.

In massage or in bathing, sweet orange oil can be used with good effect as part of a programme of general detoxifying. It will also help in the treatment of fluid retention.

Sweet orange makes a pleasant and refreshing addition to room vaporizers and blends well with other citrus fragrances and also with longer-lasting fragrances such as sandalwood.

Used in massage, sweet orange also acts to the benefit of the digestive system, toning a sluggish digestion, stimulating peristalsis and gently easing problems of constipation and flatulence. It can also help combat the problems of fluid retention and mood changes that are associated with premenstrual syndrome.

In bathing, massage or inhalation, sweet orange oil will soothe away anxiety and stress and encourage a more positive and optimistic attitude.

Suitable methods of use

Bathing, compresses, inhalation, massage, skin care, vaporizer/diffuser.

Precautions
None. Sweet orange oil is very safe generally. Cases of sensitization are extremely rare, but avoid exposure to the sun immediately after use to be on the safe side.

PALMAROSA – *Cymbopogon martinii var. martinii*
The plant
Palmarosa is a relative of lemongrass and citronella, coming from the same plant family, *Gramineae*. It is also related to gingergrass – *Cymbopogon matinii var. sofia* – which is used to obtain an oil that is similar but considered by most to be inferior in quality. The plant grows wild in India and Pakistan. It is now cultivated for commercial purposes in India and in Indonesia, the Comoros Islands, East Africa and Brazil, all of which produce the oil. The plant has fragrant grassy leaves.

The oil
The oil is obtained from the leaves of the plant, either fresh or dried, by the process of steam distillation. It is pale yellow or green in colour and has a sweet floral smell. Palmarosa essential oil is used in the perfume industry as a fragrance ingredient. It is also used in the production of soaps and bath products.

Essential oil of palmarosa is useful in the treatment of stress-related feelings of depression. It calms troubled spirits and lifts the mood, encouraging a more optimistic view of life.

The oil can be used in the treatment of various digestive problems, combating infection and improving digestion. It can stimulate a poor appetite and can help the intestinal flora to return to a state of balance after a bout of infection or following antibiotic treatment. Use in massage or in bathing.

Palmarosa oil is very useful in skin care, where its balancing qualities make it suitable for the treatment of a variety of conditions, either associated with dry or oily skin. It helps regulate the production of sebum and also moisturizes dry skin. It can be used to good effect on mature complexions, reducing wrinkles and improving the skin's tone and appearance. It will also help reduce scar tissue. Use in facial massage, creams or in facial steam baths.

Suitable methods of use
Bathing, compresses, inhalation, massage, skin care, vaporizer/diffuser.

Precautions
Palmarosa is quite safe to use in dilution. It is nontoxic, nonsensitizing and nonirritant.

PARSLEY – *Petroselinum sativum*
The plant
Parsley is either grown as a biennial or a perennial, although the latter will not live for many years. It is native to the Mediterranean area, but now grows extensively throughout Europe and in parts of Asia. Parsley is a member of the plant family *Apiece* (*Umbelliferae*). In Great Britain, it is a very popular garden herb with many culinary uses. For the purposes of oil production, it is cultivated in countries that include Germany, Holland and France.

Parsley is high in vitamins A and C. In herbal medicine, it is used for problems of the kidneys and urinary tract and also in the treatment of arthritis. Parsley is pleasant to chew on as a breath deodorizer after spicy or garlicky food. It is also a digestive aid.

The oil
Essential oil of parsley is obtained by steam distillation of the plant. Two different oils are obtained – one from the seed and one from the foliage. Parsley oil is used to treat cystitis and other urinary infections. It also acts as a diuretic. It is an emmenagogue so can be used to treat scanty and irregular menstruation.

Massage with oil of parsley can aid digestion, having a carminative and stimulating effect. Parsley oil is also used in the treatment of arthritis and rheumatism. Owing to its possible toxicity if used inappropriately, however, parsley is not recommended for use at home.

Precautions
Warning: Not recommended for home use. Parsley oil can be toxic unless used in strict moderation. It is also a skin irritant. **Warning:** Not to be used during pregnancy. Parsley oil is an emmenagogue.

PATCHOULI – *Pogostemon cablin*
The plant
Patchouli belongs to the family *Lamiaceae* (*Labiatae*) and is tall, bushy herb with large aromatic leaves. It is native to tropical Asia. It is cultivated for commercial

use in Asia, India, China and South America. The plant has white flowers and the leaves are hairy in texture. The plant has been widely used in Asia for many years as an incense ingredient. The leaves were used in woven materials to perfume them. Patchouli is also used as an insect repellent.

In herbal medicine, particularly in China and Japan, patchouli is used to treat colds, headaches and digestive upsets, including vomiting.

The oil

Essential oil of patchouli is obtained by the process of steam distillation from the leaves of the plant which are previously dried and fermented. The oil is thick and viscous and is orange-amber in colour. It has a distinctively sweet and earthy smell that is long-lasting and, unlike that of other essential oils, actually improves with age, although the fragrance of patchouli oil is not to everyone's liking – some people dislike it intensely. Patchouli oil is used in the manufacture of perfumes and soaps and is an ingredient in Indian ink.

Patchouli oil has various therapeutic applications. It is antiseptic and anti-inflammatory and can be used in skin care to treat acne, oily skin and open pores as well as minor sores that are weeping and reluctant to heal. It is also beneficial in the treatment of athlete's foot, chapped and painful skin and eczema. Patchouli is particularly beneficial to ageing skin and will also help prevent scars and stretchmarks.

When used in a massage blend, particularly in abdominal massage, or alternatively in a warm compress, patchouli can relieve constipation and combat flatulence.

In massage oil or in room vaporizers, patchouli oil is an effective room deodorizer. Used in this way, it can also be used to strengthen the spirits when exhaustion has set in and will help restore a sense of calm and determination in stressful times. The oil also has aphrodisiac properties and can benefit in particular those whose desire or sexual performance has been adversely affected by stress and fatigue.

Patchouli oil can also be used as an insect repellent.

Suitable methods of use
Bathing, compresses, inhalation, massage, skin care, vaporizer/diffuser.

Precautions
None. Patchouli oil is nontoxic, non-sensitizing and nonirritant.

PEPPERMINT – *Mentha piperita*
The plant
There are several different varieties of mint: peppermint and spearmint are the two that are used in aromatherapy. Peppermint is a perennial herb, a cultivated hybrid grown all over the world. It is easy to grow and spreads rapidly from underground runners. Some gardeners find this aspect of an otherwise useful herb rather irritating. The peppermint plant is bushy, growing to approximately 3 feet (0.9 metres) in height, has soft, fragrant green leaves and small, white flowers. Peppermint belongs to the plant family *Lamiaceae* (*Labiatae*). Peppermint is grown commercially for

production of its essential oils in several countries, including England, France, Italy and Russia. Peppermint is one of the oils for which an organic option is easily available.

Peppermint has a long history of use in herbal medicine. There is evidence that the herb was used by the ancient Egyptians, and in various countries it has been used as a treatment for various complaints, including indigestion, colic and flatulence, nausea (in particular during pregnancy), headaches and sore throats. The herb is often drunk in an infusion, as peppermint tea.

The oil

Essential oil of peppermint is produced by the process of steam distillation. The herb is harvested while in flower and the leaves, stems and flowers are used in the process. Peppermint oil is pale greenish-yellow and has a strong, fresh minty smell. Essential oil of peppermint is widely used as a flavouring ingredient in the food and drinks industries and by the cosmetics and pharmaceutical industries as a flavouring and/or fragrance in toothpastes, soaps, mouthwashes, bath products, perfumes and colognes.

Peppermint oil has various therapeutic uses and can be used to treat disorders of the respiratory system and the digestive tract as well as musculo-skeletal pain, in addition to being a valuable oil to use in skin care.

The anti-inflammatory and analgesic properties of the oil can benefit muscular pain and neuralgia, particularly when used in massage. Peppermint oil will also help to stimulate the circulation.

The anti-inflammatory properties of peppermint oil can also help to ease the irritation of pruritis when used in bathing.

Peppermint oil is astringent and will be of particular benefit to oily skins. It is, however, irritating to some sensitive skins and should be used in dilution of no more than 1 per cent in a massage blend. Three drops are quite sufficient for bathing.

As a digestive aid, essential oil of peppermint works effectively in massage to stimulate a sluggish digestion, to relieve dyspepsia and nausea and also to ease stomach cramps and colic.

Used in steam inhalation, peppermint oil has a marked anticatarrhal and expectorant action and can do much to relieve colds and bronchitis. In a mouthwash, it can deodorize bad breath.

Peppermint oil refreshes the mind as well as the body and will help to lift the spirits, give courage and focus and clear muddled thoughts.

Suitable methods of use
Bathing, compresses, inhalation, massage, mouthwashes, skin care, vaporizer/diffuser.

Precautions
Nontoxic and generally nonirritant if used in appropriate dilution. A small chance of sensitization in some individuals. **Warning:** Avoid during pregnancy. Do not swallow mouthwash.

PETITGRAIN – *Citrus aurantium var. amara* (*see also* NEROLI and ORANGE (BITTER))
The tree
The bitter orange tree, or Seville orange, as it is also known,

is indigenous to the Far East but now grows extensively in Mediterranean countries, where it is also produced commercially. It is an evergreen tree, a member of the plant family *Rutaceae*, with bitter tasting dark coloured oranges and fragrant blossom. Neroli is obtained from the blossom of the tree and bitter orange oil from the fruits. Petitgrain was originally obtained from the fruits when they were unripe and still very tiny, like little grains, hence the name of this oil, but is now produced from the leaves and twigs of the tree. France and Paraguay are two of the main sources of the highest quality oil.

The oil

The oil is produced from the leaves and twigs of the tree by the process of steam distillation. It is pale yellow to orange-amber in colour and smells pleasantly fresh, fruity and woody. As with neroli, bitter orange oil and also sweet orange oil, petitgrain can be used in the treatment of anxiety, stress and insomnia. It is very soothing and calming, whether used in massage, bathing or in a vaporizer.

Petitgrain works to the benefit of a sluggish digestive system, easing the discomfort of symptoms such as dyspepsia and flatulence. Petitgrain is similar in its effects to neroli and can be used as a less expensive alternative if neroli is prohibitively costly.

Like the other orange-based oils, petitgrain has a toning and astringent effect on the skin, refreshing a tired complexion and combating oiliness. It also acts as an antiperspirant.

Petitgrain is used in the cosmetic and pharmaceutical industries as a fragrance ingredient in the manufacture of various toiletries, colognes and perfumes. It is an ingredient in classic eau de Cologne.

Suitable methods of use
Bathing, compresses, inhalation, massage, skin care, vaporizer/diffuser.

Precautions
None. Petitgrain is very safe to use.

PINE, SCOTS – *Pinus sylvestris*
The tree
Pinus sylvestris, more commonly known as Scots pine, is a tall evergreen native to Britain where it was long ago the main species in the Great Forest of Caledon, covering much of Scotland. Now the Scots pine is grown worldwide and is cultivated commercially in several countries, including Austria, the countries of Scandinavia and the United States. Scots pine belongs to the family *Pinaceae*. There are other varieties of pine that are cultivated for their oils, for example longleaf pine and dwarf pine, but Scots pine is the one most commonly used in aromatherapy.

In herbal medicine, young pine shoots were used in bathing to treat several complaints, including rheumatism, poor circulation, skin problems and nervous fatigue. They were also used in steam inhalation for a variety of respiratory disorders. Pine was much appreciated for its insecticidal properties and was used around the house to repel parasites.

The oil
The essential oil is obtained from the needles of the tree by

the process of dry distillation. It is colourless generally but can be tinged with yellow. The oil has a strong, clean, balsamic smell. The fragrance of pine oil makes it a strong favourite in the production of many soaps and other bath products. It is also used extensively as an ingredient in household cleaning products and disinfectants as well as in insect repellents.

Therapeutically, oil of pine is versatile and quite a safe oil for home use. Its effects are refreshing and stimulating. It is particularly useful in the treatment of many respiratory ailments, such as bronchitis, influenza, coughs, colds and also asthma. It is an effective expectorant and is also antiseptic, antiviral and bactericidal. It can be used to treat respiratory tract infections either by massage or in inhalation. Steam inhalation is particularly beneficial as the steam helps to loosen excess mucus in the airways and unblock the sinuses.

Pine oil is valuable in the treatment of urinary tract infections, particularly when used in baths or sitz baths. Its antiseptic and antimicrobial properties combat infection while the patient's spirits are soothed by the refreshing fragrance.

Hot compresses of pine and massage with essential oils both work well to relieve the aches and pains of disorders such as arthritis, rheumatism and gout. Pine oil also benefits poor circulation. It is a good oil to use in the treatment of post-illness fatigue or exhaustion brought on by stress, replacing tension with relaxation and fatigue with refreshment.

Pine oil used in a room spray, vaporizer or diffuser will disinfect the air, creating a fresh and healthy atmosphere.

Suitable methods of use
Bathing, compresses, inhalation, massage, skin care, vaporizer/diffuser.

Precautions
Pine oil is generally safe to use. It is nontoxic and generally nonirritant, provided that it is used in dilutions of less than 2 per cent. A small minority of people may become sensitized. Avoid using pine on people who already have allergic skin conditions. **Warning:** Some therapists recommend that you avoid using essential oil of pine during the first three months of pregnancy.

ROSE – CABBAGE ROSE – *Rosa centifolia*, and DAMASK ROSE – *Rosa damascena*
The plant
There are two main varieties of rose that are used for the production of essential oil for aromatherapy. *Rosa centifolia*, or cabbage rose, and *Rosa damascena*, damask rose. Cabbage rose, also known as French rose, rose de mai or rose maroc, is believed to have come originally from Persia but is now cultivated commercially, mostly in Morocco and France. The plant is approximately 8 feet (2.4 metres) in height and produces a mass of fragrant pink blooms. Damask rose, also known as Turkish rose and rose otto, is thought to be indigenous to China but is now cultivated mainly in Bulgaria and France for its oil. It is a smaller plant, which also produces abundant pink blooms. Of the two varieties, cabbage-rose oil is more widely available for aromatherapy use. Rose otto can be prohibitively expensive.

Roses were widely used medicinally in ancient times in the East for a variety of ailments, which included fever, skin problems, digestive and circulatory problems. They

were also valued for their aphrodisiac properties. Symboli-
cally, the rose signifies love and has done so for many hundreds of years. Rose hips are still valued highly for their
nutritional value: they are particularly high in vitamin C.

The oil

Steam distillation of rose petals is sometimes used to produce essential oil of rose, and for many years the principal
method of extraction favoured by the perfume industry was
enfleurage. Essential oil of rose is extremely expensive, however, and an alternative is the absolute. First, a concrete is
obtained through solvent extraction of the rose petals and
then, once the solvent has been removed, the absolute is sepa-
rated from the concrete using alcohol.

The essential oils of both cabbage rose and damask rose
are yellow in colour, while the absolutes are deeper in hue,
being orange-red. The absolute is almost solid at room temperature, becoming liquid when the bottle is held and gently
warmed in the hand. Both essential oil and absolute have a
rich, deep, sweet floral smell. Beware of imitations: synthetic copies of rose oil abound and it is also quite frequently
adulterated before being sold.

Rose oil is extensively used in the perfume industry. Being
an ingredient of more than a third of the fragrances. It is also
used in the manufacture of toiletries and cosmetics and sometimes as a flavouring agent. Rose water – a by-product of
the steam distillation process – is used in cookery and for
cosmetic purposes.

Rose oil is a pleasant and safe oil to use in aromatherapy
and is suitable for a variety of uses. It is expensive, but its
strength ensures that one or two drops added to a blend will

transform it. Cabbage-rose oil and damask-rose oil have similar properties and effects.

Rose oil relaxes and strengthens, imparting a feeling of calm and wellbeing. It is beneficial to use in times of stress and will bring relief to many stress-related conditions, soothing frustration and irritability and lifting the spirits. It can be used to good effect on children and is enjoyed by most people in massage blends or in bathing. Rose oil is also delightful to blend with other essential oils in a vaporizer.

In the treatment of gynaecological problems, rose oil can be particularly beneficial. It is useful in the treatment of premenstrual tension and in menopausal difficulties such as heavy menstrual bleeding. Its effects are balancing, and it can also help to regulate infrequent or scanty menstruation. Like jasmine, rose oil has aphrodisiac qualities and can benefit both sexes by increasing libido.

Rose oil can also benefit the respiratory system and can be used to treat coughs and allergy-related respiratory complaints.

The effects of rose oil on the digestive system are detoxifying, anti-inflammatory and strengthening. It can be used to treat constipation and nausea and is also thought to have a tonic effect on the liver and gall bladder.

Rose oil is an extremely valuable oil for skin care. It is anti-inflammatory and soothing, which makes it suitable for the treatment of dry and itchy skin, and it will also help to tone a tired complexion. It is suitable for use on sensitive and ageing skin.

Rose oil also has a beneficial effect on the circulation.

It is important to point out that although rose oil is very

costly, a little of this intoxicating fragrance goes a long way in a blend.

Suitable methods of use
Bathing, inhalation, massage, skin care, vaporizer/diffuser.

Precautions
Safe to use; nontoxic, nonirritating and non-sensitizing.
Warning: Use of rose oil during early pregnancy is not advisable unless under the supervision of a trained aromatherapist.

ROSEMARY – *Rosmarinus officinalis*
The plant
Rosemary, symbol of remembrance, originally comes from the Mediterranean area but is now grown worldwide and is cultivated for oil production in France, Spain and Tunisia. Rosemary is a member of the plant family *Lamiaceae* (*Labiatae*). It is a relatively easy herb to grow and is popular as a flavouring ingredient in the cookery of many countries. It is also a favourite in scented gardens and herb gardens. Planted alongside a path, where the leaves will give off their delicious fragrance every time someone brushes past the plant, rosemary is a delight to grow. The herb grows as a small bushy shrub with grey-green aromatic leaves, like needles, all along the stem. The flowers of the plant are small and pale greyish blue in colour. Rosemary has been used in herbal medicine for centuries and also had considerable religious and spiritual significance in some countries. It was believed in several cultures to give protection against evil

spirits. In medieval times it was used as a fumigating agent against the plague. The herb has been used to treat respiratory, digestive, skin and nervous complaints and is still recommended as a general stimulant. Rosemary was also used as a treatment for depression and general debility. The stimulating effects of the herb on the mind and body have long been appreciated.

The oil

Essential oil of rosemary can be extracted from the whole plant by steam distillation, but a better quality oil is obtained if only the young leaves and flowering tips are used. The oil is either pale yellow or colourless and has a fragrance that is strong, fresh and herbal. The fragrance of the oil does not, however, closely resemble that of the plant itself. Rosemary oil is used extensively in the perfume and cosmetics industries, in the manufacture of soaps, shampoos and other toiletries and in perfumes and colognes. It is also used in the production of many food and drink products.

The effects of essential oil of rosemary are warming, stimulating, strengthening and toning, both on the body and the mind. It is thus a good all-round tonic oil to use and has many therapeutic applications.

Rosemary has particular benefits for the circulatory system. Used in a bath or in massage it will stimulate a poor circulation and relieve the discomfort of cold extremities.

Rosemary oil can be used to good effect in bathing, massage or adding fragrance to a room to stimulate the mind, helping concentration, improving memory and relieving mental fatigue: 'Rosemary for remembrance'. (It is interesting to note that the ancient Greeks wore sprigs or garlands of rosemary at times when they wanted to achieve this effect.)

Rosemary is a good oil to use in massage or bathing both before and after strenuous exercise. It is therefore invaluable to have in the house if there are athletes, walkers or cyclists in the family. It will help to tone the muscles and help prevent against strain before exercise. Following exercise, it will soothe aches, pains and stiffness. Rheumatism and arthritis can also be relieved by using rosemary oil, which is soothing and warming either in massage and bathing or with the use of compresses applied to the affected areas of the body.

The pain-relieving properties of essential oil of rosemary also make it useful in the treatment of headaches, and its stimulating properties help to restore concentration and revitalize the spirits, particularly when fatigue from overwork has set in.

The stimulating effects of rosemary will work for the benefit of the digestive system, and it can be used to treat flatulence, colic and an irritated colon. Abdominal massage can be particularly beneficial. Massage with rosemary oil also has a detoxifying effect on the body, stimulating lymphatic drainage.

Rosemary oil is antiseptic and antimicrobial and can be used in the treatment of colds, influenza and bronchitis. Use in steam inhalation or, for a comforting warming effect all over, in bathing or massage. It can also be used in a mouthwash to combat oral and throat infections. When used as a room fragrance, rosemary gives off a delicious aroma while at the same time disinfecting the atmosphere.

Rosemary oil is a popular oil to use in hair care. It can be applied in a massage blend rubbed into the scalp and can be used to treat hair lice and scabies. It also counteracts greasy hair, seborrhoea and dandruff and it may also be of benefit in some cases of hair loss (alopecia).

In skin care, rosemary oil is particularly beneficial for oily skins that are prone to spots as it is antiseptic and astringent.

Suitable methods of use
Bathing, compresses, hair care, inhalation, massage, mouth-wash, skin care, vaporizer/diffuser.

Precautions
In the correct dilution, rosemary oil is generally safe to use. **Warning:** Should be avoided during pregnancy. Not suitable for use by sufferers of epilepsy or high blood pressure.

ROSEWOOD – *Aniba rosaedora*
NOTE
Rosewood has been harvested for years without any programme for replacing the trees with new plantings. This has been very damaging environmentally. Rosewood is slow-growing and resources are becoming increasingly limited. The rainforests have suffered greatly as a consequence of the felling of the trees for timber and oil. Those who have any regard for the environment will probably choose not to use this oil, in spite of its therapeutic benefits, unless given proven assurance that the oil comes from a sustainable source. Many (and most reputable) suppliers of essential oils will also refuse to sell the oil unless it meets environmentally conscious criteria.

The tree

The tree is a tropical evergreen of medium size and grows in the Amazon basin. It is a member of the family *Lauraceae*. The timber has been used for many years in the production of high-quality furniture and is also exported to Japan for the manufacture of chopsticks. Peru and Brazil are the largest producers of rosewood oil.

The oil

The essential oil of rosewood is obtained from wood chippings by the process of steam distillation. The oil is colourless or pale yellow and has a sweet, pleasantly woody fragrance. Rosewood oil was formerly used as a source of linalol for the perfume industry, but now most linalol is synthetic. Rosewood oil is still used in the manufacture of perfumes and perfumed products and is also extensively used in the food and drinks industries.

Therapeutically, rosewood is balancing, calming, uplifting and toning. It is a sensual oil to use in massage or in a vaporizer to scent a room, and it blends well with a variety of different oils, in particular the citrus and floral oils. It can help to relieve tense headaches, soothe stress and aid concentration.

Rosewood oil is antiseptic and antimicrobial, and it strengthens the body's immune response. It can be used in massage, bathing or inhalation to help combat influenza and similar infections. It has reasonably good expectorant properties and can help to soothe dry coughs. Not only will rosewood oil help the body to fight off troublesome infections, it will also make sufferers feel better in themselves and can help combat the depressive symptoms that are often associated with a severe bout of influenza.

In skin care, rosewood oil can be used for a variety of purposes. It is anti-inflammatory and will soothe dry, sore complexions. It is widely appreciated for treating ageing skins, scarring, dermatitis and eczema.

Suitable methods of use
Bathing, compresses, inhalation, massage, skin care, vaporizer/diffuser.

Precautions
None. Rosewood oil is nontoxic, non-sensitizing and nonirritant.

SANDALWOOD – *Santalum album*
The tree
Sandalwood, a member of the family *Santalaceae*, is native to India where it is now cultivated for commercial purposes, particularly in the southern state of Karuataka, formerly known as Mysore. The sandalwood tree is a small evergreen, a parasite that gets nutrients from photosynthesis but draws the water and minerals that it requires from the roots of a host tree. (Mistletoe belongs to the same family.)

There has been some concern over depleting resources in recent years, but this problem is now being resolved with replanting programmes that have been initiated by the Indian government, which also regulates the quality of the oil that is produced. Another variety of sandalwood, Australian sandalwood, is also used for essential oil production but the Indian sandalwood is considered superior and is thus the one of choice.

Sandalwood has been used for its perfume for some four thousand years in the East. In powdered form it is burned as incense and it has been used as a component in the embalming process. Its ceremonial and religious uses include weddings, funerals and festivals. It was also used therapeutically in Eastern traditional medicine for fighting off disease.

The wood was used for building and for ornamental carvings, in particular for temples.

The oil

Sandalwood oil is obtained from the heartwood of the tree, which has previously been dried and powdered, by steam distillation. It is used as a perfume and a fragrance fixative in cosmetics, aftershaves, colognes and perfumes. It is one of the essential oils that appeals equally to both sexes. Sandalwood oil is a component of many varieties of incense. It also has value as a flavouring in some commercially produced food and drinks.

Sandalwood oil is safe to use in massage, bathing, skin care and inhalation. It will do much to relieve anxious feelings of depression. It has a relaxing, soothing effect on the spirits. It is cooling, quietening and calming and is often used by those who meditate. Sandalwood oil can help break the vicious circle of insomnia, wherein the sufferer has trouble sleeping, becomes anxious about not sleeping and then finds it even harder to sleep because of the anxiety. Sandalwood will induce a state of relaxation that is conducive to sounder, easier sleep.

The skin can benefit from the use of sandalwood oil as an emollient and anti-inflammatory agent on dry, cracked and tender skin. It cleanses and softens and is pleasant to apply in dilution to the face after shaving. It is also mildly astringent. Its fragrance has an almost universal appeal. Sandalwood is also valued for its aphrodisiac properties and is believed to increase sexual enjoyment, in particular for men.

Used in the bath, sandalwood oil is extremely beneficial to the genito-urinary system and can help in the treatment of vaginitis, leucorrhoea, cystitis and urethritis. It is anti-inflammatory and antiseptic and can also be used to treat some sexually transmitted diseases.

Used in steam inhalation, sandalwood can help in the treatment of dry coughs and heavy, mucousy colds. It is an effective decongestant and can help to clear catarrh.

Suitable methods of use
Bathing, compresses, inhalation, massage, skin care, vaporizer/diffuser.

Precautions
None. Sandalwood oil is nontoxic, non-sensitizing and nonirritant.

STAR ANISE – *Illicium verum*
The tree
Native to southeast China, the tree is a medium-sized evergreen, growing up to 40 feet (12 metres) in height. The fruits are star-shaped, with between five and thirteen seed pockets radiating from the centre. The tree, a member of the *Illiciaceae* family, also grows in India and Japan. The main source of the fruits and oil is China although some star anise is exported from India as well.

Star anise has a long history of use in traditional Chinese medicine, where it has been used as a digestive aid, an antispasmodic and for the treatment of coughs for thousands of years.

The oil

The essential oil of star anise is produced from the fruits by steam distillation. The oil is clear or tinged with yellow and smells very sweet, rather like liquorice. It is effective at masking other less pleasant tastes and smells and is used extensively by the pharmaceutical industry as a flavouring ingredient, especially to render certain medications more palatable. It is also used as a fragrance ingredient in various toiletries and as a flavouring in the manufacture of a number of foods and beverages.

Therapeutically, star anise is a sedative oil and is valued for its soothing, relaxing properties. It is a useful oil to use in massage or vaporizers to achieve a comforting sense of calm.

Star anise is particularly beneficial to the digestive system, for the relief of distressing symptoms such as hiccups, flatulence, stomach cramping, colic and indigestion. It can be used in massage blends for this purpose and massaged gently over the stomach and abdomen.

In steam inhalation, star anise oil is an effective expectorant so helps clear excess mucus from the airways. and also does much to soothe coughs and colds.

In general massage or in compresses the oil will relieve muscle cramping and can also be used to treat joint and muscle stiffness and aches and pains.

Star anise has very similar properties to the oil that is distilled from the herb aniseed, but as aniseed is a dermal irri-

149

tant and not recommended for home use, star anise is a safer alternative, provided that it is well diluted. It is not recommended, however, for bathing.

Precautions
Warning: Use star anise well diluted (2 per cent dilution or less) and in moderation as it can have a narcotic effect. Star anise oil an cause irritation in some individuals with damaged or very sensitive skin. Otherwise, it is nonirritant if used in appropriate dilution and is safer to use than aniseed, from which a similar essential oil is extracted.

TARRAGON – *Artemisia dracunculus*
The plant
Tarragon is a perennial herb native to Europe, Siberia and Mongolia. It is now grown all over the world and is a popular culinary herb, particularly in France, which is one of the main sources of the essential oil. Other producers include Holland and the United States of America. The name *dracunculus* means 'little dragon' and in France, tarragon is known as *herbe au dragon*, or the 'dragon herb'. It is a member of the family *Asteraceae* (*Compositae*).

Tarragon grows well in sunny situations but can be damaged by frosts in winter. It grows to a height of approximately 2 feet (0.6 metres) and the slender aromatic leaves are dark green in colour. The flowers are small and yellow. Two varieties are cultivated: Russian and French.

In ancient times, the herb was used as an antidote for various poisonous animal and insect bites. The root of the plant was also used to treat toothache. In Persia, tarragon was eaten to stimulate the appetite.

The oil
Essential oil of tarragon is obtained by the process of steam distillation from the leaves of the plant. The oil is either colourless or pale yellow in appearance. It has a strong, spicy smell, fresh and green in quality. It is used for its fragrance in the manufacture of toiletries and perfumes, and for its flavour it is extensively used by the food and drinks manufacturing industries.

Therapeutically, tarragon has a stimulating effect on the digestion. It is also antispasmodic and can relieve hiccups, flatulence and colic. Tarragon has therapeutic value in the treatment of some menstrual dysfunctions. The effects of the oil on the circulation is stimulating. However, tarragon oil has a degree of toxicity and is not recommended for home use.

Precautions
Warning: Not suitable for home use. Avoid during pregnancy.

TEA TREE – *Melaleuca alternifolia*
The tree
Tea tree grows as a shrub or small tree in Australia. It is a member of the family *Myrtaceae*. Its leaves are slender, like needles, and the flowers are either yellow or purple in colour.

The leaves of the tree have a very long history of use by the aboriginal people of Australia, who used them to make an infusion for drinking – hence the name 'tea tree'. The leaves were also used, crushed, for application to wounds and sores. The properties for which the tree has been appreciated for many hundreds of years make the essential oil of tea tree one of the most exciting and versatile oils in aromatherapy.

The oil
Tea-tree oil is extracted from the leaves of the tree by steam distillation. It is pale yellow-green in colour and has a strong, spicy and pleasant odour reminiscent of camphor. It is used very extensively in the pharmaceutical and cosmetics industries in the manufacture of antiseptic and germicidal preparations, gargles, toothpastes, bath products and skin treatments. Organically produced tea-tree oil is now widely available.

Tea-tree oil is one of the most useful oils in aromatherapy – many would claim it is the most useful. It is safe to use, it can be applied neat to the skin, and it has powerful antiseptic, disinfectant, antiviral, antifungal and bactericidal properties, which make it of value in the treatment of a wide variety of ailments. It also stimulates the body's immune response against infection. Tea-tree oil is a 'must' for the first aid kit.

The immuno-stimulant, antiviral and bactericidal properties of tea-tree oil make it particularly beneficial in the treatment of colds and influenza and other respiratory tract infections. For this purpose, steam inhalation is recommended. Alternatively, use the oil in a massage blend. For throat infections and painful mouth infections, for example oral thrush, gingivitis and ulcers, tea-tree oil can be used in mouthwashes and gargles. It is also effective in combating bad breath and can be used to treat cold sores.

For treating genito-urinary infections, such as cystitis, thrush, herpes, pruritis and urethritis, tea-tree oil can be used in a bath, or a sitz bath. It is very soothing and will combat infection.

In the area of skin care, tea-tree oil can be used to good effect for the treatment of a wide variety of problems. It can be used in facial steam treatments, lotions and massage blends for the skin. It can be dabbed neat onto spots and blemishes, insect bites, minor burns and stings. It is antiseptic and will also bring relief from discomfort. It can be used to treat fungal skin infections such as athlete's foot and ringworm. Leg wounds and ulcers that are difficult to heal, particularly if the sufferer is elderly and has poor circulation, can benefit from treatment with tea-tree oil in a bland carrier such as almond oil.

Research continues into the therapeutic applications of tea-tree oil and there is optimism that there are still further benefits to be derived from its immunostimulant and antimicrobial properties.

Suitable methods of use
Bathing, compresses, inhalation, massage, mouthwashes, skin care, vaporizer/diffuser. Can be applied neat to the skin.

Precautions
Tea-tree oil is nontoxic and nonirritant. There is a small chance of sensitization in a few individuals, but this is rare.

THYME, COMMON – *Thymus vulgaris*
The plant
Common thyme is a member of the plant family *Lamiaceae* (*Labiateae*). There are many varieties of thyme. Common

thyme is derived from wild thyme. It is native to, and grows extensively in, the area around, the Mediterranean. The plant is low-growing and shrub-like with small white or pale blue/purple flowers and has aromatic leaves. It also grows in other European countries and in North Africa, and it is popular in many countries as a culinary herb.

The herb has been used therapeutically since ancient times. The Greeks burnt it to fumigate buildings against infectious disease. It was also a symbol of courage to the ancient Greeks. The ancient Egyptians used thyme in the process of embalming. The Romans used it to flavour cheese.

In herbal medicine, thyme is used in combination with other herbs for the treatment of various gastric and respiratory ailments and for fever.

The oil

Two different oils are produced from the herb. The first is red thyme oil, which is obtained by steam distillation from the leaves and flowers of the plant. The second, white thyme oil, is produced after a second distillation process has been carried out. Red thyme oil, as its name suggests, is brownish red in colour. It has a strong, spicy, warm smell. White thyme oil is very pale yellow in colour and smells sweeter and less pungent than red thyme oil. Red thyme oil is much stronger and more of an irritant than white thyme oil; the latter, therefore, is safer to use.

Thyme oil is used extensively in the pharmaceutical industry, in the manufacture of antiseptic mouthwashes, toothpastes, throat lozenges, disinfectants, etc. The cosmetics industry uses it as a fragrance ingredient in soaps, shampoos and bath products.

Thyme oil is a powerful antiseptic and germicide. It also has a stimulating effect on the nervous system. It can, however, irritate the skin and should only be used well diluted. In bathing, a dilution of only 1 per cent is recommended.

Thyme oil can be used to treat respiratory infections such as colds, influenza and bronchitis, either in steam inhalation or in massage. It also has beneficial effects on the respiratory system if used in a vaporizer. It is an expectorant so also helps relieve spasmodic coughing. An added benefit of thyme oil is its immunostimulant properties, which help the body to fight off infection. Used in a vaporizer, diffuser or room spray with other antiseptic oils it will help to disinfect the atmosphere in a sick-room.

Thyme oil can be used to treat a variety of infections of the genito-urinary tract, including cystitis and urethritis.

Used in massage in particular, thyme oil can bring relief from the symptoms of arthritis and rheumatism and will also combat the stiffness and aches that are associated with over-exertion and sports-related muscle strain. It also benefits the circulatory system with its stimulating effects and can combat low blood pressure.

Provided that it is well diluted, thyme oil can be used in skin care for a variety of purposes. It can benefit oily skin and acne and has been shown to be effective against lice and scabies.

The effects of thyme oil on the nervous system are stimulating: combating mental fatigue, nervous debility and symptoms of stress such as headaches.

Suitable methods of use
Bathing, compresses, inhalation, massage, vaporizer/diffuser

Precautions
Use with care. Dilute well. Do not use on broken or sensitive skin. **Warning:** Not suitable for children, epileptics or those who are prone to high blood pressure. Avoid the use of thyme oil in pregnancy.

VETIVER – *Vetiveria zizanoides*
The plant
Vetiver is a grass, a member of the family *Poaceae* (*Gramineae*) and it is native to southern India, Sri Lanka and Indonesia. It grows to a height of approximately 6 feet (1.8 metres). It has deep, strong roots and is planted in some countries to protect the soil from erosion. It is now cultivated in several countries, including India, Reunion, Java, Haiti and Brazil.

Vetiver roots have been used for hundreds of years for their fragrance and the grass is used for weaving mats.

The oil
The essential oil of vetiver is produced from the roots by steam distillation. Vetiver oil is used extensively in the perfume industry and in the manufacture of scented toiletries. It also has uses in the food industry. The essential oil is reddish dark brown and has a woody, earthy smell that is almost musty. It is quite viscous and benefits from being gently warmed in the bottle before it is used, to make it flow more freely. The oil has a strong odour (that may not be to everyone's taste) and should be well diluted to avoid it being too overpowering in a blend.

Therapeutically, vetiver oil has a profoundly relaxing effect on the nervous system, relieving tension and stress. It can be used to good effect in the treatment of insomnia. In India, vetiver oil is known as 'the oil of tranquillity'.

In baths or in massage, vetiver is beneficial in the treatment of the symptoms of disorders such as arthritis, rheumatism and aching, stiff muscles. It is warming and comforting and will help to relieve the tension that is often associated with chronic pain.

Vetiver oil also benefits the circulatory system, stimulating and warming, especially when used in combination with massage.

In skin care, the antiseptic and slightly astringent properties of vetiver can be used to good effect in the treatment of oily skin that is prone to spots.

Suitable methods of use
Bathing, compresses, inhalation, massage, skin care, vaporizer/diffuser.

Precautions
None. Vetiver is nontoxic, non-sensitizing and nonirritant.

YLANG YLANG – *Canaga odorata var. genuina*
The tree
Ylang ylang is indigenous to Indonesia, the Philippines, Java and Madagascar. Madagascar is one of the main sources of the essential oil, which is also produced in Reunion and the Comoro islands. The tree grows to a height of approximately 65 feet (19.8 metres), and it is from the large yellow or pink fragrant flowers of the tree that the oil is extracted. The yellow

flowers are considered superior to the pink ones for purposes of oil extraction.

The flowers have a long history of use in skin care and in the prevention of infection. The aphrodisiac properties of the flower have been appreciated for many hundreds of years, and in Indonesia ylang ylang blooms were traditionally scattered on the beds of newly-wed couples on their wedding night.

The oil

The flowers are steam distilled to produce the essential oil. A total of four distillations take place. The product of the first distillation is known as ylang ylang extra and is the most expensive and the highest quality. The three following distillates, known as grades I, II and III, are progressively diminished in complexity and quality. Ylang ylang oil was an ingredient of macassar oil, which was very popular in Victorian times as a treatment for the scalp, stimulating hair growth. The oil is pale yellow and has a powerful sweet, floral fragrance that has a hint of spiciness. It is similar in many respects to jasmine oil.

Ylang ylang oil is used extensively in the perfume industry and also in the manufacture of cosmetics, soaps and toiletries. Ylang ylang extra is the oil sought after for high quality perfume production.

Ylang ylang has many uses in aromatherapy. It has a sedative effect on the nervous system and will calm anxiety and help with problems of insomnia. It will help relieve feelings of depression, especially if these are stress induced. Because of the strength of the fragrance, which can become overpowering and in some cases can cause headaches and/or nausea, ylang ylang is best used well diluted.

In bathing, room perfuming or in massage, particularly in sensual massage, the aphrodisiac properties of the oil can be used to good effect, encouraging relaxation and enjoyment.

Ylang ylang also benefits the circulatory system and can calm palpitations and help to lower raised blood pressure. It will also help to treat hyperpnoea (excessive breathing after exercise).

In skin care, ylang ylang can soothe insect bites and will have a balancing effect on the skin, making it beneficial in the treatment of acne and oily skin as well as dry skin.

Suitable methods of use
Bathing, massage, skin care, vaporizer/diffuser.

Precautions
Generally safe to use – nontoxic, non-sensitizing, nonirritant. Can cause headaches and nausea if used in strong dilutions.

NOTE
Ylang ylang can be used in the treatment of high blood pressure and tachycardia, but if you suffer from these, you should seek qualified advice regarding treatment. Both can be symptoms of more serious disorders.

Aromatherapy and Pregnancy

Aromatherapy can play a very important part in helping a mother-to-be cope with the demands that pregnancy places upon the body. Massage and relaxation will do much to help a tired and anxious expectant mother care for herself and for the new life inside her. Aromatherapy can also play a part in the birth itself, both in pain relief and relaxation as nature takes its course. After the birth, of course, the mother finds herself in a whirl of feeding and bathing and changing the baby, waking several times during the night. It can be hard, trying to keep calm and energized with the demands that a small baby can make, but once again, there are ways in which aromatherapy can make things easier for both mother and child.

It must be remembered, however, that the body is in a state of great change during pregnancy and also that treating a pregnant woman is much the same as treating two individuals: the woman and the tiny baby she carries inside her.

Some oils must be completely avoided during pregnancy as they can be harmful for different reasons – some are, in fact, abortifacients. Others are less hazardous but many therapists will nevertheless recommend that their use is avoided.

When using essential oils for massage or bathing during pregnancy, use half the quantity of oil to base that you would normally use.

Oils to be avoided during pregnancy
Throughout pregnancy, the following oils should be avoided:

aniseed
basil
cedarwood
citronella
clary sage
clove
coriander
dill
fennel
hyssop
juniper
marjoram
myrrh
nutmeg
parsley
peppermint
rose (unless on the advice
of a trained therapist)
rosemary
tarragon
thyme

In addition to the above, it is recommended that these oils are avoided in the first three months of pregnancy:

cajeput
chamomile
eucalyptus
lemongrass
melissa
niaouli
pine

lavender
(this oil is generally very safe but some aromatherapists
recommend that it is avoided in early pregnancy

There is quite a variety of literature devoted to the subject of aromatherapy during pregnancy and childbirth. Whilst much of the literature is very useful, anyone who is embarking upon the great adventure of pregnancy, whether for the first time or not, would be well advised to consult a professional aromatherapist for additional personal advice. Every person and every pregnancy is different. You stand to gain greater benefit and more reassurance from taking individual advice from an expert. Both you and your baby deserve it.

Aromatherapy and Children

Babies

Babies are highly responsive to touch and to smell from the moment of birth onwards, and there is a great deal of benefit to be derived, both for the mother and for the child, from the use of massage and aromatic oils.

Very new babies should not be treated with essential oils but can be massaged gently with almond oil or olive oil. Make sure the baby is warm and comfortable before you start, and stroke the child's body and limbs gently and rhythmically. If the baby seems unduly fretful then discontinue the process. It is unlikely to be the massage that is causing the child's distress, but little is to be gained from persisting if the child is unable to relax because of discomfort or hunger.

Once the baby is four weeks old, you can start to introduce essential oils and use them twice or three times a week. Chamomile and lavender are quite safe to use in the appropriate dilution: at this stage, use one drop of essential oil to one tablespoonful of carrier oil, no more. Take great care to keep the oil away from the baby's face. After a few months you can introduce other oils: mandarin, neroli and rose are generally considered suitable.

You can also place a bowl of hot water with a couple of drops of essential oil in the baby's room: mandarin or lavender will be particularly soothing and fragrant. If the child has a cold, you can put a drop of eucalyptus oil in a bowl of hot water close to the cot to help clear a snuffly nose.

As is the case with pregnancy, you will be able to find a great deal of literature on the subject, but for both your and the baby's benefit and for your own peace of mind, your first step should be to consult a professional.

Young children

A wider variety of oils may be used on children as they grow older. Never use oils that are known to be possible skin irritants on children, however. From when the baby is one year old onwards, you can use two drops of essential oil per tablespoon of carrier. From when the child reaches the age of around six or seven years, you can use half the quantity of essential oil that you would for an adult. Normal adult doses can be used after the age of twelve or thirteen.

Home Selection:
Preferred Essentials

As you become familiar with different oils and more expert at blending them for personal use, you will, needless to say, build up your own stock for use in the home. There are some oils, however, which are particularly useful to have in the house at all times.

Citronella
Citronella has many therapeutic applications and its deodorizing and insect-repellent properties make it particularly useful to have in the house.

Eucalyptus
Eucalyptus oil is an essential standby, especially in the winter when coughs and colds lurk everywhere, waiting to strike. It can be used in a vaporizer, both to treat respiratory infections and to disinfect the room. It is a valuable oil to use in steam inhalations for respiratory problems and it will also do much to ease stiffness in muscles and joints when used in massage.

Grapefruit
Fresh and fragrant, grapefruit oil is energizing and detoxifying and particularly useful for times when tiredness and overindulgence strike and you are feeling bloated and sluggish. If you need a fresh start, you need grapefruit oil.

Jasmine/ylang ylang

Jasmine oil is very expensive, so if you find the price prohibitive, you may prefer to use ylang ylang. These two oils have been chosen for inclusion in the list of preferred essentials primarily for their luxurious, sensual, feel-good qualities. We all deserve something like this from time to time.

Lavender

Lavender oil is invaluable. As first aid for burns and stings and for the treatment of a variety of skin problems it is extremely useful to have in the house. It is also soothing and calming and makes a relaxing and pleasingly scented addition to massage or bath blends. It also can be used to treat several respiratory and digestive ailments.

Mandarin

If you have children, mandarin oil is a useful essential oil to keep in stock. Its soothing, calming properties will come in useful when they are fretful and 'overwound' and its pleasantly fruity fragrance is almost universally popular. If you don't have children, it is still worth keeping in store for your own benefit. We all get overwound sometimes, after all.

Rosemary

Rosemary oil is a wonderful tonic for the body and the mind. Keep it in the house for use in baths and massage blends to relieve muscle and joint stiffness, soothe headaches, banish mental fatigue and boost flagging spirits. It can also be used in skin care and in the treatment of respiratory complaints.

Tea tree

Like lavender oil, tea tree is a first-class first aid oil to have in the house. Its antiviral, antibacterial and fungicidal properties make it suitable for the treatment of a wide variety of complaints, particularly of the skin, the respiratory system and the genito-urinary system.

Massage

There are several forms of therapy that make use of different forms of massage: reflexology, shiatsu, Swedish massage, physiotherapy and sports treatments to name a few. Aromatherapy makes extensive use of massage in treatment, and aromatherapists study the specific techniques involved in detail, along with anatomy and physiology, when they are training.

Origins of massage

We massage ourselves nearly every day. The natural reaction to reach out and touch a painful part of the body – such as a sprain – forms the basis of massage. As long ago as 3000 BC massage was used as a therapy in the Far East, making it one of the oldest treatments used by humans. In 5 BC in ancient Greece, Hippocrates recommended that to maintain health, a massage using The therapeutic value of applying oils and rubbing parts of the body to lessen pain and prevent illness was recognized among the ancient Mediterranean civilizations. In ancient times scented oils were almost always used when giving massages, creating an early form ofaromatherapy massage.

Swedish massage

Swedish massage, which dates from the nineteenth century, is widely used by the beauty industry and uses techniques of kneading, rolling and squeezing the flesh and effleurage (*see* massage techniques page 178). It is a relaxing form of massage and helps to improve the circulation and boost lymphatic drainage.

Aromatherapy massage is not quite the same as Swedish massage, but employs some of the same techniques. Swedish massage is quite safe and the techniques involved can be used, if desired, in the application of essential oils at home.

Swedish massage is a combination of relaxing effects and exercises that work on the joints and muscles, but it is still based on the form that was practised in ancient times. More recently, a work was published in the 1970s called *The Massage Book*, by George Downing, and this introduced a new concept in the overall technique of massage, that the whole person's state should be assessed by the therapist and not solely the physical side. The emotional and mental states should be part of the overall picture. Also combined in his form of massage were the methods used in reflexology (*see* page 197) and shiatsu (*see* page 245), and this was known as therapeutic massage. The aim of this is to use relaxation, stimulation and invigoration to promote good health.

Uses
Massage is commonly used to induce general relaxation, so that any tension or strain experienced in the rush of daily life can be eased and eliminated. It is found to be very effective, working on the mind as well as the body. It can be used to treat people with hypertension (high blood pressure), sinusitis, headaches, insomnia and hyperactivity, including people who suffer from heart ailments or circulatory disorders. At the physical level, massage is intended to help the

body make use of food and to eliminate the waste materials, as well as stimulating the nervous and muscular system and the circulation of blood. Neck and back pain are conditions from which many people suffer, particularly if they have not been sitting correctly, such as in a slightly stooped position with their shoulders rounded. People whose day-to-day work involves a great deal of physical activity, such as dancers and athletes, can also derive a great deal of benefit from the use of massage. Stiffness can be a problem that they have after training or working, and this is relieved by encouraging the toxins that gather in the muscles to disperse. Massage promotes a feeling of calmness and serenity, and this is particularly beneficial to people who frequently suffer from bouts of depression or anxiety. Once the worry and depression have been dispelled, people are able to deal with their problems much more effectively and, being able to do so, will boost their self-confidence.

Medical use
Physiotherapy and sports medicine
Massage in physiotherapy and in sports medicine tends to concentrate on specific areas of the body where there is muscle strain or injury. It tends to be used as a localized treatment for a localized effect, being its aim remedial rather than relaxing. It is therapeutic, like aromatherapy massage, but unlike aromatherapy massage it is used for treating a part of a person rather than a whole being. Neuromuscular massage, a technique that uses relatively heavy pressure compared to other forms of massage, is used with other techniques in sports therapy. Mechanical devices may also be used in sports massage. Therapeutic massage of this sort is

best left in the hands of those who have been specifically trained.

An aid to recovery

In hospitals, massage has been used to ease pain and discomfort as well as being of benefit to people who are bedridden, since the flow of blood to the muscles is stimulated. It has also been used for those who have suffered a heart attack and has helped their recovery. A more recent development has been the use of massage for cancer patients who are suffering from the after-effects of treatment, such as chemotherapy, as well as the discomfort the disease itself causes. Indeed, there are few conditions when it is not recommended. However, it should not be used when people are suffering from inflammation of the veins (phlebitis), varicose veins, thrombosis (clots in the blood) or if they have a raised temperature such as occurs during a fever. It is then advisable to contact a doctor before using massage. Doctors may be able to recommend a qualified therapist, a health centre may be able to help or contact can be made with the relevant professional body.

Psychological benefits

Along with the diagnosis element of massage there are great psychological benefits – the enjoyment of touch and of being stroked and caressed by another person. During a massage the patient is coaxed from emotional and occupational stresses and brought into the intense arena of the here and now. The importance of this kind of one-on-one nonverbal communication can never be underestimated in our increasingly impersonal and detached society.

Massage has a wide range of uses for a variety of disorders. Its strengths lie in the easing of strain and tension and inducing relaxation and serenity, plus the physical contact of the therapist. Although doctors make use of this therapy in conjunction with orthodox medicine, it is not to be regarded as a cure for diseases in itself and serious problems could occur if this were the case.

Physical benefits
Massage affects the whole body through rhythmically applied pressure. Gentle pulling and stroking movements increase the circulation of the blood and cause the blood vessels to dilate. The stimulation of nerves and blood will also affect the internal organs. Lymph is a milky white liquid that carries waste substances and toxins away from the tissues via the lymphatic system. Inactivity can cause an unhealthy build-up of this substance, and as the circulation of the lymph is largely dependent on muscle contractions, so massage will help speed the lymph's progress through the system. Active people can also benefit from massage as strenuous activity burns up the muscle, producing an increase of waste products in the muscle tissue. Massage will help to balance the system in both cases and can increase oxygen capacity by 10–15 per cent.

By realigning our bodies, massage can go a long way to repairing our generally damaged postures. Inactive lifestyles and sedentary occupations have created a society of people with cramped, stooped and neglected postures. Not only does massage help to coax the spine and corresponding physiology back into position, it also makes us more aware of our bodies. Relieved of muscle tension, the body feels lighter and can therefore be borne more naturally and with more poise. Used in conjunction with postural therapies such as Pilates or the Alexander technique, massage can help achieve a relaxed yet controlled posture.

Women in labour have found that the pain experienced during childbirth can be eased if massage is performed on the buttocks and back. The massage eases the build-up of tension in the muscles, encouraging relaxation and easing of labour pains. It is said to be more effective on women who had previously experienced the benefits and reassurance of massage.

Many of the benefits of massage come through the healer/patient contact. Our hands are one of the most sensitive parts of our body, and we experience much of our sense of touch through our hands. An experienced masseur is able to use his or her hands to communicate feelings of harmony and relaxation. A practised masseur will also be able to diagnose the patient through touch. He or she can 'listen' to tension and stress through the texture of the skin, knotted muscles and stiff joints. Old and current sprains, congestion and swelling should all be obvious to a good masseur. The actions of massage – the stroking, kneading and pulling – detoxify the body, improving circulation and lymphatic drainage. After tension and weaknesses in the body have been pinpointed and relieved, the patient is left feeling, relaxed and energized.

The massage session
Preparation
A session may be undertaken in the patient's home, or he or she can attend the masseur or masseuse at a clinic. At each

session the client will undress, leaving only pants or briefs on, and will lie on a firm, comfortable surface, such as a table that is designed especially for massage. The massage that follows normally lasts from 20 minutes to one hour.

If performed by professionals, massage is not a technique for the unduly modest. It achieves best results if the person receiving the massage is either naked or else dressed in the scantiest of underwear. For anyone who is competent and wishes to provide some simple massage for a partner, there are some basic rules to follow. The room should be warm and peaceful. People will find it difficult to relax if they are cold, and the person performing the massage will be faced with a mass of goose pimples. The surface on which the person lies should be quite comfortable but firm. Use a mid-thigh level table or the floor. A futon (a quilted Japanese mattress) can be used, and to relieve the upper part of the body from any possible discomfort, a pillow should be placed underneath the torso. Any pressure that may be exerted on the feet can be dispelled by the use of a rolled-up towel or similar placed beneath the ankles. Both people should be relaxed, and to this end soft music can be played. All the movements of the hand should be of a continuous nature. It is suggested that the recipient always has one hand of the masseur or masseuse placed on him or her. Should the masseur or masseuse get out of breath, he or she should stop for a rest, all the while retaining a hand on the person.

Aromatherapy massage

Although it is the usual practice for an aromatherapist to give whole-body massage, it will often be the case that specific areas of the body are given particular attention if required. For example, aching muscles in the back or tension in the shoulders and neck can be given specific treatment during the course of the massage procedure. At home, if free time is limited and a full-body massage is out of the question at any particular moment, great benefit can still be gained from more localized massage to 'problem' areas. A soothing abdominal massage using appropriate oils can do much to help when digestion is sluggish or when periods are painful. A shoulder and neck massage will smooth out knots of tension and help to relax the subject. If a whole-body massage is not convenient or practicable, then a careful foot massage will benefit not only the feet but the whole person. The principles of reflexology and aromatherapy are quite compatible and indeed many aromatherapists use reflexology in the treatment of their patients. The added bonus of reflexology is that foot massage can quite easily be carried out by individuals on themselves. There are many helpful books on the topic for those who are interested.

A variety of techniques will be used by the professional aromatherapist. As in Swedish massage, kneading and effleurage will be used quite extensively, but in addition to this some deep pressure can be employed, for example in the specific area of muscle pain, and attention will be paid to the meridians of the body to allow energy to flow freely and help the body to restore harmony within itself. The massage will be 'tailored' to the individual's needs, just as much as the choice of the oils that are used. Whether the overall effect of the massage is stimulating, relaxing or balancing will depend upon what is required.

Those who have visited a professional aromatherapist will attest to the fact that they feel quite different when the treatment is finished. The oils generally take around twenty to thirty minutes to take effect so their benefits will already be being felt by the time the massage is complete, and the effect of the oils, combined with massage, can be quite astonishing. Those who are visiting an aromatherapist for the first time may be advised to leave the car at home: a deeply relaxing massage can make the subject very sleepy.

Aromatherapy massage at home
Precautions
Massage is generally quite safe, but there are certain circumstances that render it inadvisable. Massage is inappropriate (and can sometimes be dangerous) if any of the following conditions are present:

epilepsy
coronary disease
fractures, open wounds, severe bruising, haemorrhage (or
   history of same), recent scarring
fever, or infectious disease with fluctuating temperature
contagious skin disease
sunburned skin
osteoporosis
high blood pressure
varicose veins
areas of acute inflammation
nausea
undiagnosed swellings or lumps

Preparation
The first thing to ensure is that you are fit to carry out the

massage. If you are suffering from back pain you cannot massage properly and you risk further injury to yourself. Similarly, it is best to massage a partner, friend or family member only if you yourself feel that you have the energy. Choose a time when you feel calm and relaxed but not tired. Ensure that you are wearing comfortable, light, loose clothing that will not hinder your movements or make you become overheated. Avoid long, wide sleeves – short sleeves are preferable – and don't wear necklaces or pendants that could dangle over the subject and cause irritation. For the same reason, if you have long hair, keep it tied back out of the way. Wash your hands thoroughly and make sure that your nails are clean and short. Before beginning massage, make sure that your hands are warm.

Ensure that the room is very warm. Lighting should be good but not too bright. Massage can be carried out on the floor, with something soft laid down for the subject to lie on, but it is easier for the person carrying out the massage if a surface such as a long table (not too high) can be used. Beds are generally unsuitable – the massage surface needs to be firm – but a thin, firm mattress placed on the floor or table will make your subject more comfortable and thus make it easier for both of you to achieve maximum benefit. Have all the oils that you might require ready to hand, and some tissues to wipe your hands on or to wipe up any accidental spillages. Soft music can be played in the background if so desired to provide additional enjoyment and a calm, soothing atmosphere. Ensure that you will not be interrupted by telephones or other people. If there are others in the house, ask them to stay out of the room and to try to keep noise down to a minimum. The latter two aims can be particularly hard to achieve when there are children in the house. Waiting until they are asleep or choosing a time when they are out of the house might be preferable.

Talk to your subject for a while to find out how he or she is feeling mentally and physically in order to allow you to prepare a massage blend that is most suitable for the moment. Make sure that at least one hour has passed since your subject's last meal. Remember that if you are new to aromatherapy, it is best to keep your blends simple. As you prepare your blend and mix it with your carrier oil, ask your subject to undress and lie on the table or floor. Cover your subject with towels and ensure, during the course of the massage, that you keep him or her covered, apart from the area on which you are working.

Massage techniques
Basic techniques
Massage can be divided into four basic forms, and these are known as percussion (also known as drumming); friction (also called pressure); effleurage (also called stroking) and petrissage (also called kneading). These methods can be practised alone or in combination for maximum benefit to the patient.

Percussion (drumming or tapotement)
Percussion is also called tapotement, which is derived from tapoter, a French word that means 'to drum', as of the fingers on a surface. As would be expected from its name, percussion is generally done with the edge of the hand with a quick, chopping movement, although the strokes are not hard.

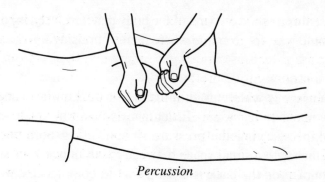

Percussion

This type of movement would be used on places like the buttocks, thighs, waist or shoulders where there is a wide expanse of flesh.

Friction (pressure)

Friction strokes are used to penetrate into deep muscle tissue. Friction is often used on dancers and athletes who experience problems with damaged ligaments or tendons. This is because the flow of blood is stimulated and the movement of joints is improved. Friction can be performed with the base of the hand, some fingers or the upper part of the thumb. It is not advisable

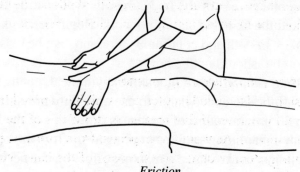

Friction

179

to use this method on parts of the body that have been injured in some way, for example where there is bruising.

Effleurage

Effleurage is widely used in massage and is quite a simple movement to carry out. Effleurage is basically a form of stroking, varying the pressure to suit, using both hands together with a small space between the thumbs (A). Using effleurage on the back is a good way to commence a mas-

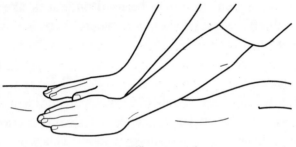

Effleurage – A

sage as it relaxes the subject and spreads the essential oils over a large surface of skin right from the start. Thus, as you work on other areas of the body, the oils will already have penetrated the skin and started to work. Begin gently, keep the strokes smooth and continuous. Pressure can be reasonably firm but should not be heavy.

Effleurage is performed in a slow, rhythmical, controlled manner. If the therapist wishes to use only light pressure he or she will use the palms of the hands or the tips of the fingers with light gliding strokes, working away from the heart. Light gliding strokes have a relaxing effect on the nervous system. For increased pressure the knuckles or thumbs will

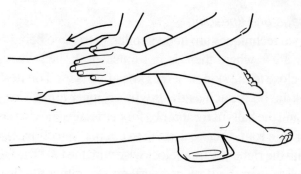

Effleurage – B

be used in an upwards stroking motion towards the heart to promote venous return. Stronger pressure has more of an effect on the blood circulation and the nervous system.

Effleurage can be used on the upper leg as far up as the hip on the outside of the leg. Once the person is lying face downwards (with support under the chest), continue to use effleurage movements on the back of the lower leg. Continue as before but work on the upper leg (B), avoiding the knee. The muscles in the buttocks can be worked upon with both hands to squeeze but making sure that the hands are moving in opposite ways (C).

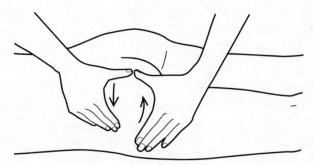

Effleurage – C

Petrissage and kneading

These two techniques are quite similar, petrissage being suitable for areas where there is not much flesh, i.e., when the bone is close to the skin, whereas kneading is used on fleshier areas of the body such as the thighs or upper arms. Use fingertips and the balls of the thumbs for petrissage, moving small areas of skin round between them in circular direction, clockwise with the right hand, anticlockwise with the left. The hands do not slide over the flesh as in effleurage; rather the flesh is moved, one small area at a time, by the fingers and thumbs.

Kneading is carried out with straight fingers and thumbs lifting an area of flesh and passing it to the other hand. Pressure can be quite firm but should not be painful.

Petrissage and kneading help to break down deposits in the tissues and stimulate circulation and lymphatic drainage, helping the body to rid itself of toxins.

Petrissage is ideal for unlocking aching or tense muscles, in particular the trapezium muscle between the neck and shoulders (A). Both hands work together in a rhythmic

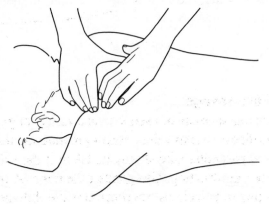

Petrissage – A

sequence, alternately picking up and gently squeezing the tense muscle. The kneading action gets deep enough to stimulate the lymph into removing the build-up of lactic acid. As the therapist works across each section, an area of flesh is grasped and squeezed, and this action stimulates the flow of blood and enables tensed muscles to relax. People such as athletes can have an accumulation of lactic acid in certain muscles, and this is why cramp occurs. Parts of the body on which this method is practised are along the stomach and around the waist (B).

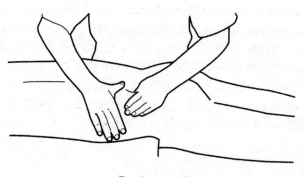

Petrissage– B

Abdominal massage
Abdominal massage can be used to treat a variety of gynaecological and digestive complaints. Heavy pressure should **never** be used and particular care should be taken if the subject is pregnant or menstruating. Use gentle effleurage (A on page 184), working in a clockwise motion round the abdomen with light strokes, aiming to relax and soothe the subject.

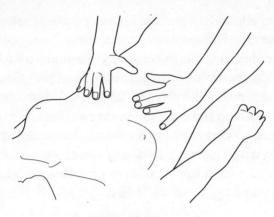

Abdominal massage– A

Another technique for the abdomen is to glide the hands across but moving in opposite ways (B).

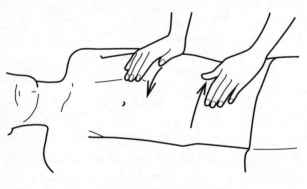

Abdominal massage– B

Back massage

When massaging the back, it is best to start with effleurage, working with one hand on either side of the spine. Work from the bottom of the spine upwards, stroking upwards and, as you reach the shoulders, outwards. The subject should find this wonderfully relaxing. This is a particularly pleasant way to spread the oil from your hands onto the patient's skin. Keeping your hands on the subject, continue round over the shoulders and down the sides of the subject towards the waist. While pressure need not be very firm, it should not be too soft as the subject might find an over-gentle touch tickly.

Working on more specific areas of the back, kneading can be used on the fleshier areas at the sides. Keep your movements smooth and flowing. As one hand leaves the subject's body, the other should remain in contact, giving the patient (remember, he or she will be face down and unable to see what you are doing) a sense of security. Work up either side of the spine using petrissage, making small, circular movements with your thumbs as you move upwards from the lumbar region towards the neck. Keep the pressure firm without being heavy-handed. You should be able to feel the subject's back relax as you do this, and any tenseness you may have noticed in the way he or she has been lying on the table should visibly reduce. As you become more practised at massage, you will be able to detect specific little knots of tension in the muscles as you work, and you can give them specific attention as required.

Menstrual pain can be treated with massage of the lower back. Use petrissage, starting at either side of the sacrum (the base of the spine above the coccyx or tail bone) and working your way outwards towards the sides of the hips. Keep your movements slow, using fairly firm pressure and moving your thumbs in fairly wide circles. Keep the rhythm of your movements steady and soothing.

Finish off a back massage with effleurage over the whole area. Leave the subject to rest for a few moments before rising.

Back massage helps to relax the whole body. The strokes

should be carried out smoothly. Applying thumb pressure to the channels on either side of the spine on the upper back will help respiratory problems. The same stroke on the lower back can relieve constipation and menstrual discomfort.

Back – A
Place your hands, facing each other, on either side of the base of the spine. Move them up the back, using your body weight to apply pressure. Take your hands round the shoulders and return lightly down the sides of the body. Repeat several times before stopping to knead the shoulders. Work on one shoulder and then the other. Repeat the movement.

Back – A

Back – B
Place your hands at waist level, with your thumbs in the hollows on either side of the spine and your fingers open and relaxed. Push your thumbs firmly up the channels for about 2 ins (6 cm), relax them, and then move them back about 1 in (2 cm). Continue in this way up to the

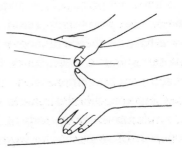

Back – B

neck. Then gently slide both hands back to the base of the spine. Repeat. Follow with the sequence in A.

Back – C
Place your hand flat across one side of your partner's back at the base of the spine. Apply firm palm pressure and work up to the shoulders. Follow closely with your other hand. Repeat using alternate hands. Work through the same sequence on the other side of the back, then repeat on both side several times. Finish by working through A.

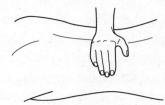

Back – C

Back – D
Place your hands, facing up the back, on either side of the spine. Applying firm palm pressure, work from the base of the spine to chest level. Turn your fingers outwards and move your hands apart to the sides of the body. Repeat this stroke at waist and hip levels. Repeat the first movement in A several times.

Back – D

Neck and shoulder massage

This can be done as part of a whole-body massage but can also be carried out when time and facilities do not permit the full treatment. It is a wonderful tension and stress reliever and can help in the treatment of tension headaches. The subject need not be lying down; he or she can sit on a chair, facing backwards, with the arms folded on the back of the chair supporting the head. A pillow placed under the arms can make this position more comfortable. If preferred, the subject can sit on a chair leaning over a table, provided that the table is high enough to avoid back strain.

Use effleurage initially, stroking in an anticlockwise direction, working round from shoulders to neck. Use petrissage on the neck at each side of the spine, working your way from the base of the neck upwards to loosen knots of tension. With the flat of your hands over the top of the subject's shoulders, work your thumbs round in circles around the fleshier area at the top of the shoulders, pushing more firmly with upwards movements of the thumbs. Finish the shoulder massage with effleurage.

Neck and shoulders – A
Stand behind your seated partner. Begin with effleurage, applying firm pressure with both hands. Start at the bottom of the shoulder blades up each side of the spine to the base of the neck. Move your hands apart across the

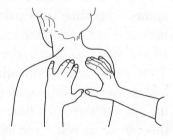

Neck and shoulders –A

top of the shoulders and then bring them gently down to the starting position. Repeat several times, finishing with a light return stroke.

Neck and shoulders – B
Stand at right angles to the side of your partner. Locate tension spots in the shoulders using your thumbs and then work these areas with the thumbs. The pressure can approach your partner's pain threshold but not exceed it.

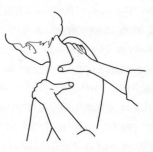

Neck and shoulders –B

Neck and shoulders – C
Place your left hand in an 'L' shape on your partner's shoulder. Applying firm pressure, move it slowly up the whole length of the shoulder. Repeat with your other hand. Continue repeating the sequence using alternate hands. Place one hand at the base of the back of the neck and move it gently up to the hairline, gently squeezing all the time. Return with a gentle

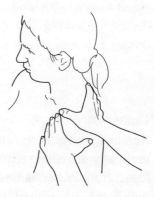

Neck and shoulders –C

stroke. Repeat several times. Without removing your hands, walk round to the other shoulder and repeat B and C. Move behind your partner and repeat A several times.

Limb massage
Leg massage
Leg massage can be wonderfully relaxing for tired and aching muscles and is extremely beneficial for stimulating a sluggish circulation. **Warning:** Varicose veins, however, should never be massaged. If you are going to carry out a leg massage, start with effleurage movements, stroking firmly upwards from foot to hip. Knead the fleshier areas of the legs, working first on the calves and then the thighs. Grip the subject's calf with your thumbs at either side of the shin and your palms, one immediately above the other, over the calf muscle, pulling gently but firmly outwards, round and back. For the thighs, work up and round with straight fingers and thumbs, moving the flesh from hand to hand, always keeping contact with the skin.

Limbs – A
Begin at the ankle and stroke vertically up the leg with one hand. Follow the same path with your other hand. Continue this sequence, using alternate hands.

Limbs – A

Limbs – B

Raise your partner's foot and hold it with the knee at a right angle. Using the palm of your free hand, stroke firmly down the back of the leg from ankle to knee level. Use a light stroke to return to the ankle. Repeat the whole movement several times. If including the foot, work through D and E next before repeating the full sequence (A to B) on the other leg.

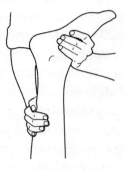

Limbs – B

Limbs – C

Help your partner to turn over, and begin by stroking with alternate hands up the whole leg, as in A. Then put your hands on either side of the knee and, using your thumbs to apply pressure, circle around the knee cap. If including the foot, bring your hands down to the ankle and use the sandwich stroke (D) on the front of the foot. Work through the full movement on the other leg.

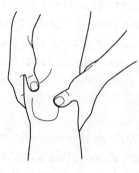

Limbs – C

Foot massage

As has already been mentioned, foot massage can be used to benefit the whole body. Foot massage has the added benefit of being an easy way to self-help in aromatherapy. Treat yourself to a warming footbath to which aromatic oils have been added, then settle down in a comfortable position in a warm room and give yourself a foot massage.

When giving a foot massage to someone else, ensure that both of you are in a comfortable position. You will probably find that unless the subject is lying on the floor or on a couch, it is best if you sit in chairs facing each other. The subject places his or her foot on a stool or low table (use something to pad the surface) immediately in front of you. It is better if your seat is slightly lower than the subject's seat.

Work all over the foot, from toe to heel with small circular movements of your fingers and thumbs. Pay particular attention to areas of discomfort or pain – these are signs of problems elsewhere in the body.

A thorough general foot massage will undoubtedly be beneficial, but further benefit will be gained if you apply the principles of reflexology which is covered in more detail in the next chapter (*see* page 197). There are many helpful books on the subject. The best way to learn is through practice, so find a book with a clear, easy-to-read chart of the reflexes on the feet and prop it up within clear sight as you massage. Initially, you may find that referring to the chart does interrupt the 'flow' of the massage somewhat, but further practice sessions will help to familiarize you with the reflexes. In time, you will be able to dispense with the chart and concentrate totally on the real foot in your hands.

Limbs – D

With your partner lying face down, take one foot between your hands, so that the palm of your upper hand is resting in the arch. Press firmly, and slowly draw your hands down to the tip of the foot. Use plenty of pressure for this 'sandwich' stoke.

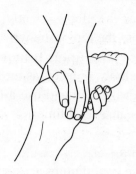

Limbs – D

Limbs – E

Hold the foot with your thumbs lying side by side behind the toes. Pull both thumbs back to the sides of the foot, then push them forward. Repeat this zig-zag movement as you work down to the heel. Then push firmly all the way back to the toes, keeping your thumbs side by side. Repeat the whole movement several times. Work through the whole sequence (D to E) on the other foot.

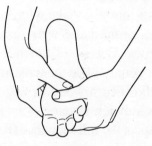

Limbs – E

Limbs – F

Take hold of your partner's hand as in a firm handshake, and lift the arm up slightly, as

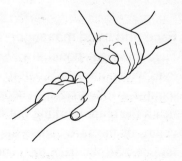

Limbs – F

193

far as the elbow. Gently place the palm of your fee hand across the top of the wrist and close your fingers round the raised arm. Apply firm pressure and slide your hand up to the elbow, or as far as the shoulder. Move your palm underneath the arm and use a light stroke to return to the wrist. Repeat several times.

Limbs – G
Place your thumbs across the inside of your partner's wrist. Applying pressure with both your thumbs, make wide circles around the wrist area. Repeat F. As you finish, relax your hold on the wrist and pull off firmly and slowly in a sandwich stroke, as in D. Repeat the full sequence (F to G) on the other arm, finishing with the hand variation of D.

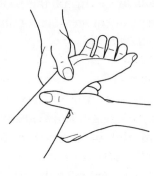

Limbs – G

Face and head massage

Face massage should always be gentle. Cover the subject's eyes with cotton pads before commencing. Using gentle effleurage, stroke from the centre of the face outwards. Start beneath the chin, working out towards the ears, then from the centre of the face across the nose, up and out towards the temples. Stroke from the centre of the forehead out towards the temples. Press more firmly at the sides of the temples and work your fingertips round in circles to ease away tension.

To improve circulation, softly tap your fingers over the subject's face, again working from the centre outwards.

The following sequence encourages deep relaxation. Gentle stroking of the forehead (B) can help to relieve stress-related tension and headaches, while pressure applied to the sides of the nose and along the cheekbones (C) alleviates nasal congestion and sinus problems. Scalp massage (D) stimulates circulation.

Face and head – A

Use alternate hands to stroke up one side of the face, starting beneath the chin and working up towards the forehead. Work through the same movement on the other side of the face. Repeat several times. Finish by placing one palm across your partner's forehead, ready for the next stroke.

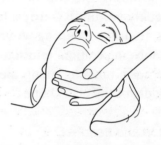
Face and head – A

Face and head – B

Begin by stroking up the forehead with alternate palms. Then place the pads of the middle three fingers of both hands in the centre of the forehead between the eyes. Draw them gently apart across the brow and round the outside corner of the eyes.

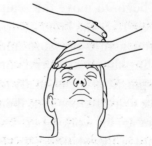
Face and head – B

Lift off the middle two fingers and use your fourth fingers only to return under the eyes towards the nose.

Face and head – C
Position your thumbs on your partner's forehead. Using the three middle fingers of both hands, press firmly against the sides of the nose. Continue along the top of the cheekbone, until you reach the temple. Keeping your thumbs in position, return to the nose, pressing along the middle of the cheekbone.

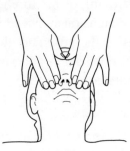

Face and head – C

Face and head – D
Spread out the fingers and thumbs of both hands and place them on your partner's scalp. Keep them in position and begin to move the scalp muscle over the bone by applying gentle pressure and circling slowly and firmly on the spot. Stop occasionally to move to a different area, then begin again, working gradually over the whole scalp.

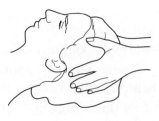

Face and head – D

Finish off the facial massage with effleurage.

Reflexology

Reflexology is gaining popularity once more in modern times, but it is an art with ancient origins, coming from the East. Reflexology works on the principle that specific zones of the body can be treated with massage of corresponding areas – reflexes – elsewhere. The foot is most commonly used for treatment, certain spots on the foot being selected for particular attention to treat corresponding areas elsewhere in the body. Reflexology, practised professionally, is not only used for treatment but also for diagnosis. Thus non-specific pain in the body that is of uncertain origin can be pinpointed quite precisely by the reflexologist upon examination and massage of the patient's foot. Reflexology is thought to be particularly beneficial in the treatment of endocrine disorders and for general stimulation of immunity and lymphatic drainage.

Origins
Reflexology is a technique of diagnosis and treatment in which certain areas of the body, particularly the feet, are massaged to alleviate pain or other symptoms in the organs of the body. It is thought to have originated about five thousand years ago in China and was also used by the ancient Egyptians. It was introduced to Western society by Dr William Fitzgerald, who was an ear, nose and throat consultant in America. He applied ten zones (or energy channels) to the surface of the body, hence

the term 'zone therapy', and these zones, or channels, were considered to be paths along which flowed a person's vital energy, or 'energy force'. The zones ended at the hands and feet. Thus, when pain was experienced in one part of the body, it could be relieved by applying pressure elsewhere in the body, within the same zone.

Subsequent practitioners of reflexology have concentrated primarily on the feet, although the working of reflexes throughout the body can be employed to beneficial effect.

Massage and energy flow
Reflexology does not use any sort of medication – merely a specific type of massage at the correct locations on the body. The body's energy flow is thought to follow certain routes, connecting every organ and gland with an ending or pressure point on the feet, hands or another part of the body. When the available routes are blocked, and a tenderness on the body points to such a closure, then it indicates some ailment or condition in the body that may be somewhere other than the tender area. The massaging of particular reflex points enables these channels to be cleared, restoring the energy flow and at the same time healing any damage.

The uses of reflexology are numerous, and it is especially effective for the relief of pain (back pain, headaches and toothache), treatment of digestive disorders, stress and tension, colds and influenza, asthma, arthritis, and more. It is also possible to predict a potential illness and either give preventive therapy or suggest that specialist advice be sought. The massaging action of reflexology creates a soothing effect that enhances blood flow, to the overall benefit of the whole body. Reflexology, however, clearly cannot be used to treat conditions that require surgery.

Reflex massage initiates a soothing effect to bring muscular and nervous relief. The pressure of a finger applied to a particular point (or nerve ending) may create a sensation elsewhere in the body, indicating the connection or flow between the two points. This is the basis of reflexology, and although pain may not be alleviated immediately, continued massage over periods of up to one hour will usually have a beneficial effect.

There are certain conditions for which reflexology is inappropriate, including diabetes, some heart disorders, osteoporosis, disorders of the thyroid gland, and phlebitis (inflammation of the veins). It may also not be suitable for pregnant women or anyone suffering from arthritis of the feet.

The best way to undergo reflexology is in the hands of a therapist, who will usually massage all reflex areas, concentrating on any tender areas that will correspond to a part of the body that is ailing. Reflexology can, however, be undertaken at home on minor conditions such as back pain, headache, etc, but care should be taken not to over-massage any one reflex point as it may result in an unpleasant feeling. Although there have not been any clinical trials to ascertain the efficacy of reflexology, it is generally thought that it does little harm and, indeed, much benefit may result.

Some practitioners believe that stimulation of the reflex points leads to the release of endorphins (in a manner similar to acupuncture). Endorphins are compounds that occur in the brain and have pain-relieving qualities similar to those of morphine. They are derived from a substance in the pituitary gland and are involved in endocrine control (glands producing hormones, for example, the pancreas, thyroid, ovary and testis).

The reflexes

Reflexes on the hands and feet

Reflexes on the feet – the soles of the feet contain a large number of zones, or reflexes, that connect with organs, glands or nerves in the body, as shown in the figures below.

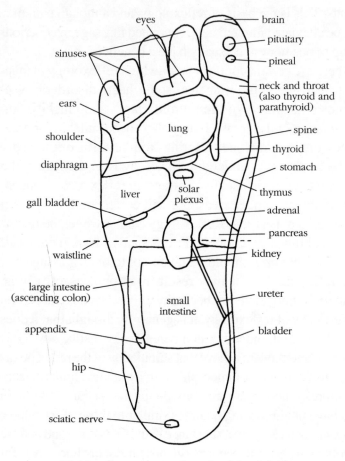

Major reflex points on the sole of the right foot

In addition, there are a small number of reflexes on the top and insides of the feet, as shown in the figures on page 202.

The *palms of the hands* similarly contain a large number of reflex areas, reflecting the arrangement seen on the soles of the feet, as shown in the figures on page 204 and 205.

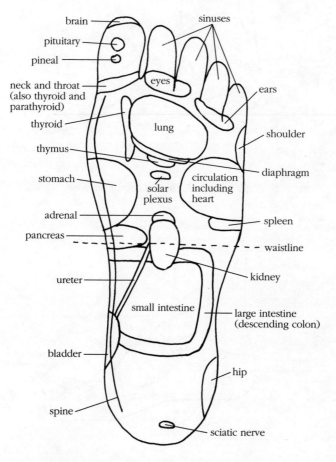

Major reflex points on the sole of the left foot

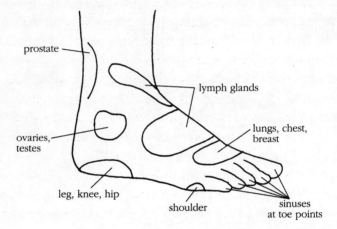

Reflex areas on the outside of the foot

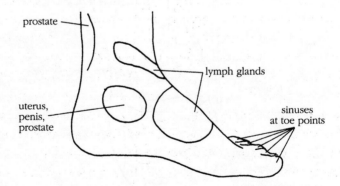

Reflex areas on the inside of the foot

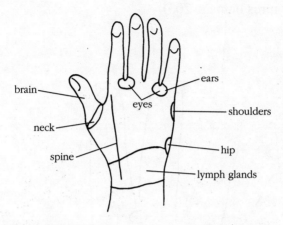

Reflex areas on the back of the right hand

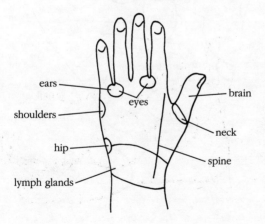

Reflex areas on the back of the left hand

The backs of the hands again mirror, to some extent, the tops of the feet, containing a smaller number of reflex areas (*see* figures on page 203).

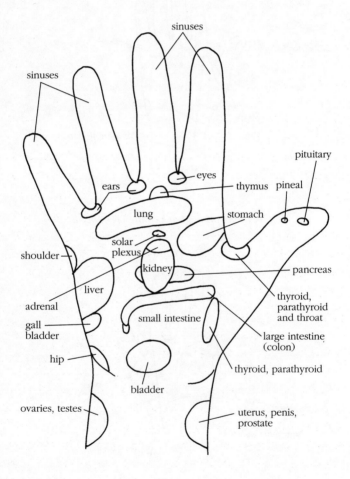

Major reflex points on the palm of the right hand

Use of the hands in reflexology

The hands are considered to have an electrical property, so that the right-hand palm is positive and the left-hand palm is negative. In addition, the right hand has a reinforcing, stimu-

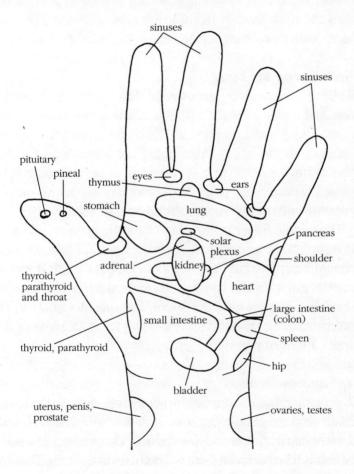

Major reflex points on the palm of the left hand

lating effect while the left has a calming, sedative effect. The back of each hand is opposite to the palm, thus the right is negative and the left is positive. This is important when using reflexology because if the object is to revitalize the body and restore the energy flow that has been limited by a blockage then the right hand is likely to be more effective. The left hand, with its calming effect, is best used to stop pain.

Reflexes on the body

Reflexes on the body necessarily differ from those on the feet and hands in that there is less alignment with the ten zones (the figures on page 207 and 208 show some of the reflexes on the body). Also, there are a number of reflex points on the body that correspond to several organs or glands. These reflex points are sometimes harder to find accurately and may be more difficult to massage.

The middle finger is thought to have the greatest effect, so this should be used to work the reflex point. Light pressure should be applied to each point, and if pain is felt it means there is a blockage or congestion somewhere. A painful point should be pressed until the discomfort subsides or for a few seconds at a time, a shorter rest being taken in between the applications of pressure.

The abdominal reflex

A general test can be applied by gently pressing into the navel, either with the middle finger or with one or both hands, with the individual lying in a supine position. The presence of a pulse or beat is taken to mean there is a problem in this area. To combat this, the same technique is used, holding for a few seconds (six or seven), releasing slightly, and keeping the fingers in the

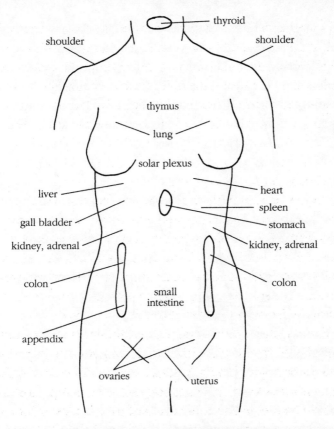

Major reflex points on the female body

same area, gently massaging with a circular action. If it is necessary to press quite deep to feel the beat, then heavier massage will be required to provide the necessary stimulation.

The same principle can be applied to other reflex points in the abdominal region, and the absence of a pulse or beat indicates that there is no problem. In each case, should there be a painful response, holding for a few seconds invokes the sedative action.

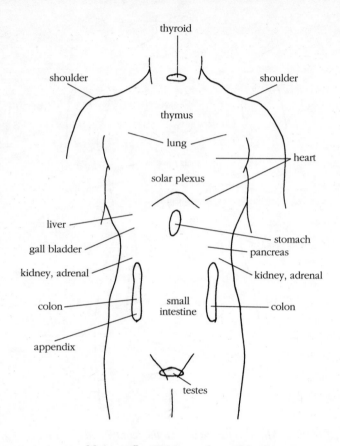

Major reflex points on the malebody

Chest reflexes

There are a number of reflex points on the chest relating to major organs in the body. The same massage technique can be adopted for these reflex points as for the abdomen. Because many of the points lie over bone or muscle, however, it will not be possible to press in the finger as deeply as for the abdomen. However, pressure should be maintained over tender areas, with a subsequent circular massage, and a similar effect will be achieved.

Reflexes on the head
There are a surprisingly large number of reflex points on the head, although all may not be apparent immediately. With

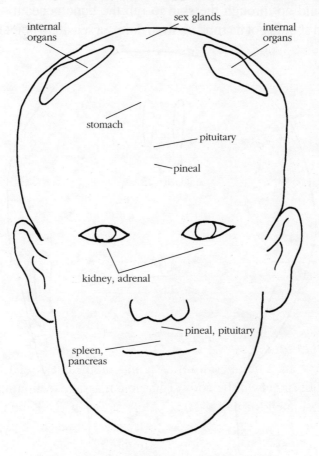

Some of the major reflex points on the head

time and experience, such points are often located more by touch than by sight.

There are many important reflexes on the head including the stomach, kidneys, spleen and pancreas. Again, the middle finger can be used for massage, beginning in the middle of the forehead with a gentle circular motion. The massage should go through the skin to rub the bone beneath – the skin should not be rubbed. In so doing, a sensitive point may

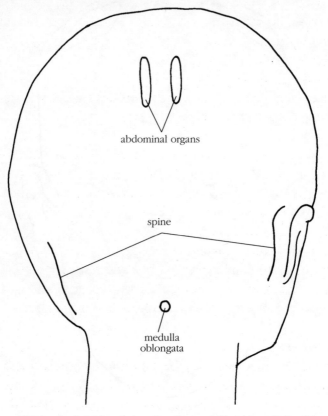

The back of the head showing the medulla oblongata reflex

be felt (pituitary) and another one a little lower down, which is the pineal. (The pituitary gland secretes hormones that control many body functions and the pineal body is thought to regulate the natural variations in the body's activities over a 24-hour period.) This massaging action can be continued to check other parts of the body.

The back of the head also shows a large number of reflexes. However, there are a number of ways of stimulating the body as a whole through the head. These include:
• tapping the head gently with the fists, all over and very quickly for a period of about thirty seconds
• pulling handfuls of hair
• tapping the head gently with a wire brush

Each has a specific result, for example, stimulating the hair, but also enlivening organs and glands over the whole body.

One particularly important reflex point is the medulla oblongata (*see* page 210). The medulla oblongata is the lowest part of the brain stem, which joins to the upper part of the spinal cord. It contains important centres for the control of respiration, swallowing, salivation and the circulation. This reflex point is located at the nape of the neck, towards the base of the skull. Massage of this point opens all channels within the body and generates a vitality, relieving nervous tension and producing almost instant energy. The point should be pressed and massaged to produce the desired effects.

Ear reflexes
The ear has long been used in acupuncture because, in addition to its ease of use, it contains scores of acupoints, which correspond to the reflex points in reflexology. Some of these points are shown in the figure on page 213.

The ear is perhaps the most difficult area of the body to work with because there are so many reflexes in such a small space. It becomes essentially a question of touch, pressing and exploring, and any sore point located can be massaged and worked out. By using a gentle squeeze-and-roll method on the tops of the ears and the ear lobes a number of areas can be stimulated. It has been reported that reflexology can help ear problems such as ringing in the ears, and the condition tinnitus may be alleviated to some extent.

Techniques and practice

Some indication of the massaging, manipulative procedures of reflexology have already been mentioned, but a number of general points of guidance can also be made.

The whole process of reflexology is one of calm, gentle movements in a relaxed state. The foot is probably used most in reflexology, in which case shoes and socks and stockings, etc, should be removed. A comfortable position should be adopted on the floor or bed, in a warm, quiet room with the back supported by pillows.

To begin, the whole foot is massaged, indeed both feet should ideally be worked on. However, if working on your own feet it is thought that the right foot should be massaged first (contrary to previous practice). It is considered that the right foot is linked with the past, hence these emotions must be released before the present and future aspects are dealt with in the left foot.

Techniques of massage vary, but a simple method with which to start involves placing the thumb in the middle of the sole of the foot. The thumb then presses with a circular and rocking motion for a few seconds before moving to an-

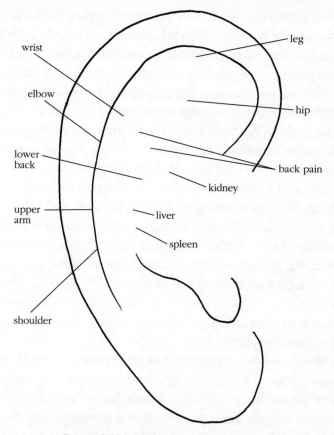

wrist

elbow

lower back

upper arm

shoulder

leg

hip

back pain

kidney

liver

spleen

Some of the major reflex points on the ear

other reflex. Reference can be made to the diagrams to determine which reflex is being massaged. In all cases, the massage should work beneath the skin, not on the skin. Another method involves starting the massage with the big toe and then moving on to each toe in turn. In using the thumbs to effect the massage, some refinements of motion can be introduced to give slightly different movements.

1 The thumb can be rocked between the tip and the ball, moving forwards over the relevant area. This, along with the circular massage already mentioned, relieves aches and pains.
2 Both thumbs can be used alternately to stroke the skin firmly. This creates a calming effect.
3 The area can be stroked with the thumbs, one moving over the other in a rotational sense. This action is intended to soothe and allow for personal development.

In addition to the procedures already mentioned, reflexology can be used to alleviate many symptoms and help numerous conditions. The following sections provide examples of these uses. Reflexology can be approached intuitively, so that the pressure of touch and the time factor can vary depending upon response and need.

The use of reflexology
The digestive system
The *stomach* is an organ that has thick muscular walls and in which food is reduced to an acidic semi-liquid by the action of gastric juices. There are many factors that can cause an upset stomach. To assess the general condition, the stomach body reflex (above the navel) can be pressed. Around it are several related reflexes such as the liver, gall bladder, intestines and colon. The reflex should be pressed for a few seconds and then released three times to activate the reflex.

On the *hands*, the web of soft tissue between the thumb and forefinger of the left hand should be worked with the thumb of the right hand for a few minutes. The hands can be reversed but the stronger effect will be gained this way, because the stomach lies mostly on the left side.

On the *feet,* the reflexes for the stomach are found primarily on the instep of the left foot, although they are also present on the right foot. These should be massaged, but there are further factors, in addition to the use of reflexology, that will aid digestion. These include eating a sensible diet with a minimum of artificial substances, and not overeating. The use of certain essential oils (aromatherapy) can also be of benefit. In this case peppermint oil can often be particularly effective.

The *colon* is the main part of the large intestine in which water and salts are removed from the food that enters from the small intestine. After extraction of the water, the waste remains are passed on to the rectum as faeces. If this system becomes unbalanced in any way, then the water may not be absorbed or the food remains pass through the colon so quickly that water cannot be absorbed. In such cases, the result is diarrhoea, which can be painful and inconvenient.

Both body and foot reflexes should be massaged for the stomach, intestines, colon and also the liver and kidneys. The thyroid reflex should also be worked to help regulation of the body functions. A useful body reflex is to press and rotate your finger about two inches above the navel for a couple of minutes. This can be repeated numerous times, each time moving the fingers a little clockwise around the navel until a complete circuit has been made.

It is important that the condition be stabilized as soon as possible as continued loss also leads to loss of vital salts and a general nutritional deficiency.

At the outset it is possible to work the colon reflexes on the hand to identify any tender areas. The right thumb should be pressed into the edge of the pad (around the base and side of the thumb) of the left palm and worked around to seek out any tender spots. Any tender reflex should be massaged and pressed for a few seconds. In each case, the tenderness should be worked out. Since there are many reflex points crowded onto the navel, it may not solely be the colon reflex that requires some attention. It is always useful to work the reflex on both sides of the body to ensure a balance is achieved.

A similar approach can be adopted for reflexes on the feet, starting at the centre, or waistline. By applying a rolling pressure, the foot is massaged along to the inner edge and then down the line of the spine and any tender points are worked through pressure and massage. It may be necessary to start with a very light pressure if the area is very tender, and then as the soreness lessens, the pressure can be increased.

Again, diet can be an important factor in maintaining the health of the body and the workings of the colon. Fibre is particularly important in ensuring a healthy digestive system and avoiding ailments such as diverticulitis.

Reflexology can be used for other conditions associated with the digestive system, notably ulcers. A peptic ulcer (in the stomach, duodenum or even the oesophagus) is caused by a break in the mucosal lining. This may be due to the action of acid, bile or enzymes because of unusually high concentrations or a deficiency in the systems that normally protect the mucosa. The result can be a burning sensation, belching and nausea.

To help alleviate the problem, which may often be stress-related, the reflexes in the feet should be massaged, as these are often the most relaxing. Obviously, the important reflexes are the stomach and duodenum, but it is also worthwhile to work on the liver and the endocrine glands (notably the pituitary). If the ulcer is a long-standing problem or if stomach complaints have been experienced for some time, then further medical help is probably needed.

The heart and circulatory system

The heart is obviously a vital organ. This muscular pump is situated between the lungs and slightly left of the midline. It projects forward and lies beneath the fifth rib. Blood returns from the body via the veins and enters the right atrium (the upper chamber), which contracts, forcing the blood into the right ventricle. From there it goes to the lungs where it gains oxygen and releases carbon dioxide before passing to the left atrium and left ventricle. Oxygenated blood then travels throughout the body via the arteries.

By using body reflexes, the heart can be maintained, and conditions can be dealt with by massaging the appropriate reflex points. A useful massage exercise is to work the muscles, rather than the reflex points, of the left arm in a side-to-side movement. This can be followed by the neck muscles and the chest muscles; in each case any tightness or tension should be massaged out. An additional preventive is a good diet, which should be low in fat and food high in cholesterol, but should contain adequate amounts of vitamins, notably the B group, C and E. Exercise is, of course, very important to maintain a good heart and circulation.

There is also a simple test that many reflexologists feel is useful in the diagnosis of possible heart problems. It may also be worth doing if strenuous activity is contemplated in the near future. Pressure is applied to the pad of the left thumb, at the top. The pressure should be quite hard. It is suggested that when this part of the pad hurts, it indicates a constriction in blood vessels, limiting supply. If the bottom of the pad hurts, this is indicative of congested arteries. If the area is too tender to touch (and there is no physical damage to the hand) then there is a possibility of a heart attack. This test thus provides advance warning and enables a medical doctor to be consulted. Should painful areas occur on both hands, this does *not* indicate a heart problem.

Many blood and circulatory disorders will benefit from the same sort of massage. In these cases the foot reflexes for the endocrine glands (hypothalamus, pituitary, pineal, thyroid and parathyroid, thymus, adrenals, pancreas, ovary or testis) should be worked well, as should those for the circulatory system and heart, lungs and lymphatic system.

Conditions that may benefit from such treatment include:

Angina
A suffocating, choking pain usually referring to angina pectoris, which is felt in the chest. It occurs when blood supply to the heart muscle is inadequate and is brought on by exercise and relieved by rest. The coronary arteries may be damaged by atheroma (scarring and buildup of fatty deposits). Of particular importance are the heart and circulatory reflexes (veins and arteries) and those of the lymphatic system.

Arteriosclerosis
A general term including atheroma and atherosclerosis (where arteries degenerate and fat deposits reduce blood flow), which results generally in high blood pressure and can lead to angina. Additional reflexes that should be worked include the liver.

Hypertension (high blood pressure)

This may be one of several types, the commonest being *essential* (due to kidney or endocrine disease or an unknown cause) and *malignant* (a serious condition that tends to occur in the younger age groups). In addition to the reflexes for the blood and circulation, those for the shoulders, neck and eyes should be worked, in combination with reflexes for the digestive system and liver.

Palpitations

An irregular heartbeat, often associated with heightened emotions. Also due to heart disease or may be felt during pregnancy. The lung and heart reflexes are particularly important, in addition to those of the circulation.

Some heart conditions are very serious and require immediate hospitalization, e.g. cardiac arrest (when the heart stops) and coronary thrombosis (a coronary artery blockage causing severe chest pain, vomiting, nausea and breathing difficulties. The affected heart muscle dies, a condition known as myocardial infarction). However, massage of appropriate reflexes may help, particularly in less serious cases. These should include the heart and circulation (veins and arteries), lungs, endocrine system and the brain. Each will have some beneficial effect in relieving stress and congestion.

Varicose veins

Veins that have become stretched, twisted and distended, and this often happens to the superficial veins in the legs. The possible causes are numerous and include pregnancy, defective valves, obesity and thrombophlebitis (the inflammation of the wall of a vein with secondary thrombosis). Phlebitis is inflammation of a vein and occurs primarily as a complication of varicose veins. Both these conditions can be treated by massaging the circulatory reflexes and also the leg and liver reflexes. In both cases, resting with the legs in an elevated position is beneficial.

The respiratory system

Asthma is one of the major problems of the respiratory system and its incidence seems to be escalating. The condition is caused by a narrowing of the airways in the lungs. It usually begins in early childhood and may be brought on by exposure to allergens (substances, usually proteins, that cause allergic reactions) exercise or stress.

There are certain body reflexes that can help in this instance. One reflex point is in the lower neck at the base of the V-shape created by the collar bones. Relief may be achieved by pressing the finger into this point with a downward motion for a few seconds. There are additional reflex points on the back, at either side of the spine in the general region of the shoulder blades. These can be worked by someone else with thumb or finger, who should press for a few seconds. Other reflexes that can be worked on the foot include the brain, endocrine glands such as the pineal, pituitary, thymus and thyroid, the lungs, and also the circulatory system. Particular attention should be paid to the lungs, which includes the bronchi and bronchioles, the branching passageways of the lungs where gaseous exchange (oxygen in, carbon dioxide out) takes place. At the point where the instep meets the hard balls of the feet, and along the base of the lung reflex area is the massage point for the diaphragm. Working the whole of this area will help alleviate symptoms of asthma. During an attack of asthma, both thumbs can be placed on the solar plexus reflexes immediately to initiate the soothing process.

The adrenal glands are found one to each kidney, situated on the upper surface of that organ. These are important endocrine glands because they produce hormones such as adrenaline and cortisone. Adrenaline is very important in controlling the rate of respiration and it is used medically in the treatment of bronchial asthma because it relaxes the airways. It is clear therefore, that the adrenal is an important reflex and it is located in the middle of each sole and palm.

Many other respiratory disorders can be helped by using massage of the same reflexes: brain, endocrine glands, lungs and diaphragm, neck and shoulders, augmented by the heart and circulatory system. Conditions responding to this regime include bronchitis, croup, lung disorders and emphysema (distension and thinning, particularly of lung tissue, leading to air-filled spaces that do not contribute to the respiratory process).

Infections of the respiratory tract leading to coughs and colds can also be helped primarily by working the reflexes mentioned above. For colds, the facial reflexes should be massaged, especially that for the nose. However, it is good practice to include the pituitary, and to work the index and middle fingers towards the tip to help alleviate the condition.

With such respiratory problems, there are complementary therapies that can help such as homoeopathy, aromatherapy and Bach flower remedies. There are also many simple actions that can be taken, for example a sore throat may be helped by gargling regularly with a dessertspoon of cider apple vinegar in a glass of water, with just a little being swallowed each time. Honey is also a good substance to take, as are onion and garlic.

The endocrine glands
Summary

Endocrine glands are glands that release hormones directly into the bloodstream, or lymphatic system. Some organs, such as the pancreas, also release secretions via ducts. The major endocrine glands are, in addition to the pancreas, the thyroid, parathyroid, pituitary, pineal, thymus, adrenal and gonads (ovaries and testes).

The endocrine glands are of vital importance in regulating body functions as summarized below:

pituitary	controls growth, gonads, kidneys; known as the master gland
pineal	controls the natural daily rhythms of the body
thyroid	regulates metabolism and growth
parathyroid	controls calcium and phosphorus metabolism
thymus	vital in the immune system, particularly pre-puberty
adrenal	control of heartbeat, respiration and metabolism
gonads	control of reproductive activity
pancreas	control of blood sugar levels

The fact that the endocrine glands are responsible for the very core of body functions means that any imbalance should be corrected immediately to restore the normality. There are some general points relating to massage of these reflex areas. It is good practice to massage the brain reflex first and then the pituitary. This is because the hypothalamus, situated in the forebrain, controls secretions from the pituitary gland. The pituitary gland then follows as this is the most important in the endocrine system. The reflexes should be gently massaged with thumb or finger for a few seconds and then gentle pressure exerted and held for a few seconds before releasing slowly.

The pituitary

An imbalance of pituitary gland secretions, often caused by a benign tumour, can lead to acromegaly (excessive growth of skeletal and soft tissue). Gigantism can result if it occurs during adolescence. There may also be consequent deficiencies in adrenal, gonad and thyroid activity. The brain and endocrine reflexes should be worked in order, supplemented by those for the circulation, liver and digestion. In addition to reflex points on the hands and feet, there is also one on the forehead. If any of these reflex areas is found to be tender, it should be massaged often to maintain the balance necessary for healthy growth.

The pineal

The pineal body, or gland, is situated on the upper part of the mid-brain, although its function is not fully understood. It would seem, however, to be involved in the daily rhythms of the body and may also play a part in controlling sexual activity. The pineal reflex points are found close to those of the pituitary on the big toes, thumbs and on the forehead and upper lip.

The thyroid

The thyroid is located at the base of the neck and it produces two important hormones, thyroxine and triiodothyronine.

Under or overactivity of the thyroid leads to specific conditions.

If the thyroid is overactive and secretes too much thyroxine (hyperthyroidism), the condition called thyrotoxicosis develops. It is also known as Grave's disease and is typified by an enlarged gland, protruding eyes and symptoms of excess metabolism such as tremor, hyperactivity, rapid heart rate, breathlessness, etc. The important reflexes on which to concentrate are the brain and solar plexus, endocrine system and also the circulatory and digestive systems. The reflexes are found on the soles and palms and using the thumbs or fingers, the areas should be massaged, but in stages if the area is very tender.

Underactivity of the thyroid, or hypothyroidism, can cause myxoedema producing dry, coarse skin, mental impairment, muscle pain and other symptoms. In children a similar lack causes cretinism, resulting in dwarfism and mental retardation. The reflexes to be worked are essentially those mentioned for hyperthyroidism, and in addition (for both conditions) the liver reflexes on the right sole and palm should benefit from attention.

There are additional thyroid reflexes elsewhere on the body, notably on the neck roughly midway between jaw and collarbone and on either side. These points should be massaged gently with the thumb and fingers on opposite sides of the throat. Using a gentle gyratory motion, the massage can be taken down to the collarbone, the fingers and thumb of the other hand are then used (on opposite sides of the throat) and the procedure repeated.

Goitre is another condition associated with the thyroid and is a swelling of the neck caused by enlargement of the gland, typically due to overactivity of the gland to compensate for an iodine deficiency. The important reflexes to concentrate upon are the brain, solar plexus, endocrine system and circulatory system but working of all body reflexes will help.

The parathyroid

There are four small parathyroid glands located behind or within the thyroid. They control the use of calcium and phosphorus (as phosphate) in the body's metabolism. An imbalance of these vital elements can lead to tetany (muscular spasms), or at the other extreme, calcium may be transferred from the bones to the blood, creating a tendency to bone fractures and breaks.

The reflexes to these glands are found in the same location as those for the thyroid but it will probably be necessary to massage more strongly to achieve an effect. It is a good idea to work on these areas each time reflexology is undertaken as they are vital in maintaining the metabolic equilibrium of the body.

The thymus

The thymus is located in the neck (over the breastbone) and is a vital contributor to the immune system. It is larger in children and is important in the development of the immune response. After puberty it shrinks although seems to become more active later in life. Bone marrow cells mature within the thymus and one group, T-lymphocytes, are dependent upon the presence of the thymus. These are important cells as they produce antibodies.

The commonest disorder associated with the thymus is myasthenia gravis, which lowers the level of acetylcholine (a neurotransmitter) resulting in a weakening of skeletal muscles and those used for breathing, swallowing, etc. The thymus reflexes are found on the soles of the feet and palms of the hand, next to the lung reflexes. The thymus can also be stimulated by tapping with the finger over its position in the middle of the upper chest.

The adrenals

The two adrenals (also known as suprarenals) are situated one above each kidney and consist of an inner medulla and an outer cortex. The medulla produces adrenaline, which increases the rate and depth of respiration, raises the heartbeat and improves muscle performance, with a parallel increase in output of sugar from the liver into the blood.

The cortex of the adrenal glands releases hormones including aldosterone, which controls the balance of electrolytes in the body, and cortisone, which, among other functions, is vital in the response to stress, inflammation and fat deposition in the body.

On both the palms and soles, the adrenal reflexes are located above those for the kidneys and if this area is at all tender, it should be massaged for a few seconds. Because the kidney and adrenal reflexes are close together, the massage should be limited to avoid over-stimulation of the kidney reflexes. Disorders of the adrenal glands should be treated by working the endocrine reflexes starting with the pituitary and including the adrenal reflexes themselves, followed by the reflexes for the circulatory, liver and urinary systems.

Specific disorders include Cushing's syndrome, caused by an overproduction of cortisone, which results in obesity, reddening of the face and neck, growth of body and facial hair, high blood pressure, osteoporosis and possibly mental disturbances, and Addison's disease, which results from damage to the cortex and therefore a deficiency in hormone secretion. The latter was commonly caused by tuberculosis but is now due more to disturbances in the immune system. The symptoms are weakness, wasting, low blood pressure and dark pigmentation of the skin. Both these conditions can be treated by hormone replacement therapy but reflexology can assist, through massage of the endocrine, digestive and liver reflexes.

The gonads

The gonads, or sex glands, comprise the ovaries in women and testes in men. The ovaries produce eggs and also secrete hormones, mainly oestrogen and progesterone. Similarly, the testes produce sperm and the hormone testosterone. Oestrogen controls the female secondary sexual characteristics such as enlargement of the breasts, growth of pubic hair and deposition of body fat. Progesterone is vital in pregnancy as it prepares the uterus for implantation of the egg cell.

The reflexes for these and related organs are found near the ankles on the inside of the feet, just below the angular bone (*see* figure depicting the reflex areas on the inside and outside of the feet on page 202). The same reflex areas are also located on the arms, near the wrist. The ovaries and testes are on the outer edge, while on the opposite, inner edge, are the reflexes for the uterus, penis and prostate.

For any disorders that might involve the ovaries or testes, it is also useful to massage other systems such as the brain, other endocrine glands, the circulation and liver.

The pancreas

This is an important gland with both endocrine and exocrine functions. It is located behind the stomach, between the duodenum and spleen. The exocrine function involves secretion of pancreatic juice via ducts, into the intestine. The endocrine function is vital in balancing blood sugar levels through the secretion of two hormones, insulin and glucagon. Insulin controls the uptake of glucose by body cells and a lack of hormone results in the sugar derived from food being excreted in the urine, the condition known as diabetes mellitus. Glucagon works in the opposite sense to insulin, and increases the supply of blood sugar through the breakdown of glycogen in the liver, to produce glucose.

The primary reflexes for the pancreas are found on the soles and palms, near to the stomach. The thumb should be used, starting on the left foot, working across the reflex area and on to the right foot. If the area is tender, it should be worked until the tenderness goes. Because there are numerous reflexes in this area, there will be stimulation of other organs, to the general wellbeing of the body as a whole.

For other disorders of the pancreas, such as pancreatitis (inflammation of the pancreas) the reflexes associated with digestion should also be worked. Pancreatitis may result from gallstones or alcoholism and, if sufficiently severe, may cause diabetes.

The liver and spleen

The role of the liver

The liver is a very important organ and is critical in regulating metabolic processes. It is the largest gland in the body and is situated in the top right hand part of the abdominal cavity. Among the functions, the liver converts excess glucose to glycogen, which is stored as a food reserve; excess amounts of amino acids are converted into urea for excretion; bile is produced for storage in the gall bladder and some poisons are broken down. The liver also recycles red blood cells to remove the iron when the cells reach the end of their life; it stores vitamins and produces blood clotting substances. Due to its high chemical and biochemical activity, the liver generates a lot of heat and is the major contributor of heat to the body.

The liver reflex points

The reflex area for the liver is a large area, reflecting the size of the organ, on the right palm and right sole, on the outer edge. As a general procedure, the area should be massaged with the left thumb, searching for tender points. More massage may be required for the liver than for other reflexes.

Hepatitis is inflammation of the liver due to viral infection or the presence of toxins. Alcohol abuse commonly causes hepatitis, and it may also be due to drug overdose or drug side effects. Viral infections such as HIV and glandular fever can also cause hepatitis. There are several types of hepatitis, designated A to E, and all may persist in the blood for a long time.

To combat such disorders, after removing the source of any toxins, the reflex for the liver and digestion should be worked and the reflexes for the eyes. Dietary restraint is also important and should involve natural foods with little or no alcohol, caffeine, nicotine and a low intake of fats.

Associated with the liver, anatomically, is the gall bladder. This is a small sac-like organ that stores and concentrates bile. When fats are digested, the gall bladder contracts, sending bile into the duodenum. Sometimes stones form here, and often gallstones can cause severe pain. The gall bladder reflex is found at the foot of the liver on the right palm and foot. On the body there is another reflex just below the ribs on the right-hand side, and below the liver reflex point. A steady pressure should be held around the point, beginning near the navel and working to the right side, maintaining pressure for a few seconds on any tender point.

The role of the spleen
The spleen is situated on the left side of the body behind and below the stomach. The spleen produces leucocytes (white blood cells), lymphocytes (a white blood cell involved in the immune system), blood platelets (involved in blood coagulation) and plasma cells. It also acts as a store for red blood cells, which are made available in emergencies (when oxygen demand is greater).

The spleen reflex point
The reflex area for the spleen is found on the left palm or sole, below the reflex for the heart. If a tender point is found in this reflex, it may indicate anaemia and it would then be wise to obtain a blood test.

The kidneys and bladder
The role of the kidneys and bladder
The kidneys are important organs in the body's excretory system. They are responsible for processing the blood continuously to remove nitrogenous wastes (mainly urea) and they also adjust salt concentrations. By testing the reflexes

with the thumb, tender areas can be located and worked upon. However, prolonged massage should be avoided – it is better to use shorter periods of 15–20 seconds initially as the system becomes accustomed to the treatment.

It is not surprising, considering the pivotal role of the kidneys in removing body wastes, that any interference with their normal function can lead to serious illnesses. General kidney disorders, kidney stones, nephritis and pyelitis are all best aided by massaging the kidney reflex but also the reflexes for the central nervous system, the endocrine glands (especially the pituitary and adrenal glands), liver, stomach and circulation. Kidney stones are formed by the deposition of solid substances that are naturally found in the urine but that precipitate out for one reason or another. They are commonly salts of calcium, and the alteration in pH of the urine is often a contributory factor. Nephritis is inflammation of the kidney and pyelitis is when part of the kidney, the pelvis, becomes inflamed. If the whole kidney becomes affected, it is then called pyelonephritis.

The kidney and bladder reflex points
Disorders associated with the bladder tend to be infections such as cystitis or other physical manifestation of a problem whether through stress or a medical condition. The latter category includes enuresis (bed-wetting) and incontinence. In these cases, the bladder reflex should obviously be worked upon, and the reflexes for the brain, solar plexus and endocrine system.

The reflexes for the kidneys are found just off centre on the palms of both hands and soles of both feet. They are close to the pancreas and stomach. The bladder reflex is towards the base of the palm, near the wrist and on the feet it is found on the inside edge of both soles, towards the heel. There are also body reflexes for both organs.

The body reflexes for the kidney are at the side of the body, almost at the waistline, between the hip and rib cage. They also occur on the face, just beneath the eyes.

The alleviation of back pain and other skeletal disorders
The reflex points for the spine
Within the working population of most countries, back pain accounts for millions of days in lost production. This is not unexpected as the spine is the primary part of the skeleton, hence any problem with it will inevitably upset the body and its overall wellbeing.

On the soles of the feet, the reflex for the spine is located along the inner edge of both feet running from the base of the big toe almost to the heel. By working this line with the fingers, any tender points can be found and worked upon. The top end of the line, near the toe, is equivalent to the spine at the level of the shoulders.

Treatment of back disorders through reflexology

With back disorders, such as lumbago, additional reflexes should be worked including the brain and endocrine system. Because the body's musculature is a complementary and antagonistic system with the skeleton, creating all the movements of which the body is capable, the muscles are also important when dealing with back pain. It will help therefore to massage muscles, rubbing quite deeply with the fingers, and moving across the muscles.

Back pain can result from a problem elsewhere in the body

with posture, tight muscles or even flat feet. It is important to be aware of the possibilities and ensure that the treatment deals with the problem as a whole, and not just in part. Exercise is clearly beneficial and walking can help loosen and strengthen muscles associated with the back. A brisk walk is fine, but jogging is not necessarily the best remedy, as in some cases this can itself prove harmful.

Reflexologists often turn to the muscles in the legs to alleviate back pain, particularly in the area of the lower back. The muscles at the back of the thigh should be massaged with a pressing and pulling action, first with one hand and then the other. The whole of the thigh should be treated, from the top of the leg, to the knee. Massage of both legs in this manner, concentrating on any 'tight' areas, will help improve the overall tone and assist in eliminating causes of back pain.

Study of the diagrams for the feet and hands reveals specific reflex areas for the shoulders, hip and neck. When working on skeletal disorders in general, it is wise to undertake a thorough massage of specific reflex areas such as neck and shoulders, plus those for the brain, solar plexus, the endocrine system, remainder of the skeletal system, endocrine glands, etc. For particular conditions such as bursitis (inflammation of a joint, as in housemaid's knee), general joint pain, stiff neck and similar complaints, a common regime of reflexological massage applies. This should include working the skeletal reflexes along with those for the nervous and endocrine system, digestive and circulatory systems. It is usually the case that the specific complaint will benefit from massage of its reflex area and most of those that comprise a whole body workout. It should always be remembered that there are occasions when surgery may prove essential, e.g. in the case of a hip replacement.

The knee joint can often be the source of pain and discomfort. It may help to apply gentle pressure on either side of the knee, just where the bone ends, using the thumb and middle finger. This should be held for a few seconds, pressing as much as possible (do not press hard if it is too painful) and then the same should be done below the knee.

Relief from arthritis with reflexology

Arthritis can be a crippling disease and many people suffer from it. It is an inflammation of joints or the spine, the symptoms of which are pain and swelling, restriction of movement, redness and warmth of the skin. Two forms of the condition are osteoarthritis and rheumatoid arthritis.

Treatment of osteoarthritis through reflexology

Osteoarthritis involves the cartilage in joints, which then affects the associated bone. What often happens is that the cartilage is lost, to be replaced by osteophytes at the edges of the bones. These are bony projections that occur with the loss of cartilage or with age. The projections affect the joint function, causing pain.

Treatment of rhematoid arthritis through reflexology

Rheumatoid arthritis is the second commonest joint disease after osteoarthritis. It usually affects the feet, ankles, wrists and fingers in which there is a swelling of the joint and inflammation of the synovial membrane (the membraneous envelope around the joint). Then follows erosion and loss of cartilage and loss of bone. At its worst, the condition can be disabling.

Massage of the reflex areas for the affected areas should be worked but, as mentioned previously, it is important to massage the reflexes for the whole body to achieve a complete and balanced approach. The endocrine system is one important system in this respect.

In seeking ways to treat rheumatoid arthritis, the medical profession isolated the glucocorticosteroid hormone, cortisone, from the adrenal glands of cattle. It was found that the use of cortisone had dramatic effects on the symptoms of rheumatoid arthritis. However, the relief was only temporary, and an additional disadvantage was the occurrence of associated side effects, which could be severe, e.g. damage to muscle, bone, stomach ulcers, bleeding and imbalances in the hormonal and nervous systems. The medical use of this compound is therefore very restricted, but it is produced naturally by the adrenal cortex. Being a natural secretion, there are no detrimental side effects. There is a reflex point in the lower back, between the first and second lumbar vertebrae, which can be pressed. Finding this point will be hit and miss initially, but upon locating it (roughly 5 cm up from the coccyx or tailbone), apply gentle pressure, gradually increasing, and hold it for a few seconds. This should be repeated several times. This is helpful for other conditions, in addition to rheumatoid arthritis, such as asthma and bursitis.

As with back disorders, muscle condition is also felt to be important in the treatment of arthritis. The muscles in the area affected by arthritis should be massaged by pressing in with the fingers, either on or near to the area. The massage should be across the muscles, with a deep motion, although it may initially produce discomfort or soreness. Many practitioners regard this as an important supplementary technique in administering reflexology.

Stress and tension
The relaxing effects of reflexology
One of the additional beneficial effects of reflexology when dealing with a particular reflex area or point is that the treatment is very relaxing. If most of the body reflexes are massaged, a feeling of wellbeing is generated, and tension is released. Stress control and relief can be accomplished in a number of ways, some of which happen instinctively, such as deep breathing and, paradoxically, wringing the hands. The latter is an obvious way of working the reflex points, albeit that it is mostly done unconsciously. A related method of calming the nerves is to intertwine the fingers, as in clasping the hands, which enables all the reflexes between the fingers to be pressed. This should be done several times. Deep breathing is a common method of relaxation that ultimately can envelop the whole body, providing that the focus of attention is the attainment of the correct pattern of breathing. Mental attitude is also an important aspect of reflexology. It clearly makes sense, while undergoing massage (with or without a practitioner or partner) to imagine, or listen to, pleasing sounds, rather than worrying about the pressures of modern life. If there is no access to relaxing sounds (bird song, running water, etc) it is perfectly possible to imagine it, and thereby to augment the physical relaxation with mental calm.

Reflex points for treating stress
The *endocrine glands* are considered important in combating stress because they are responsible for the hormonal

balance of the body. All reflex areas for these glands, on both soles and palms, should be massaged and special attention given to the thyroid, which controls body temperature and can help restore calm. The adrenal reflex point, almost in the centre of the hand, is also important, and, because it is so near the solar plexus, receives equal attention. (The solar plexus is a network of nerves and ganglia in the sympathetic nervous system concerned with body functions not under conscious control. It is located behind the stomach).

Quite often stress and tension can result in a sore neck or back. A number of reflex points can be worked to relieve these sorts of complaint. The medulla oblongata is important in this respect as it controls some major body functions such as the circulation. The point on the back of the head (*see* the figure on page 210) should be held with the middle finger for a few seconds and then released, and repeated several times. The reflex points of the spine should also be worked starting at the neck reflex, which is found below the base of the big toe or thumb. By moving down the side of the foot, the whole spine can be covered. To relieve a sore back completely and effectively, other reflexes to be attended to should include the shoulders, hips, and the sciatic nerve. The sciatic nerve is made up of a number of nerve roots from the lower part of the spinal cord, and pain with this origin may be felt in the back of the thigh, buttock and the foot. The reflex point may at first be painful to the touch, but through careful massage it can be worked to assist in promoting relief.

Control of the heart rate is a natural, complementary procedure in promoting stress relief. If a situation, wherever it may be, results in you feeling stressed, massaging the reflex areas for the heart will help, whether on foot or hand.

Sound, restful sleep is refreshing and also contributes to a reduction in stress. Reflexology can also help in this respect through the feeling of relaxation that it induces. The clasping of the hands, mentioned earlier, can be used to combat sleeplessness. The fingers can be clasped on the chest and then worked over each other so that the length of each finger is massaged. The fingers should remain intertwined and simply be released a little to allow each finger over the first knuckle, when the fingers are squeezed together again. This, associated with deep breathing will encourage relaxation.

Reflexology and the reproductive system
Reflex points for the reproductive system
The major reflexes of the reproductive system are those for the uterus, ovary and breast in the female, and the penis, testes and prostate in the male. The ovary reflexes are found on the outer side of the foot, just below the ankle (*see* figures on page 202). On the hand, these are found a little way beyond the wrist (*see* figures on page 203), on the outer edge. On both foot and hand, the breast reflex is found on the outer edge, a little below the base of the little toe or finger. The uterus reflex on the hand occupies a position opposite to the ovaries, i.e. just below the wrist, but on the inner edge of the arm. On the foot, this reflex mirrors that for the ovary, but it is on the inside of the foot, below the ankle.

The male reflexes
The male reflexes occupy the same positions as those of the female, thus the penis reflex is in the same position as that for the uterus and the testes is the same as the ovaries. The prostate gland reflexes are situated with the penis reflex and

also at the back of the leg/foot, above the heel, (*see* the figures on page 202).

There are also reflex points on the head for the gonads (*see* sex glands on the diagram of the reflex points on the head on page 209). As well as working the various reflexes for the reproductive system, it is beneficial to pay attention to the endocrine gland reflexes as they have considerable control over the gonads (*see* endocrine glands, page 222). In particular, the pituitary, thyroid and adrenal glands and their hormonal secretions have a large influence on the reproductive system. All these points should be massaged to stimulate activity and ensure that hormone secretion is balanced and gonad activity is normal. The body reflexes can also be used to this end by pressing each point for a few seconds and repeating several times for all endocrine and sex glands.

If any of the endocrine glands are tender, it may be indicating a problem with the sex glands. By working the various reflex points, it is possible to ensure a healthy reproductive system. There are a number of reflexes to the penis and testes that can help in this respect. The sex reflex below the navel should be pressed with fingers or thumb and massaged for a few seconds. Additional reflex points on the legs, about 15 cm above the ankle on the inside of the leg, should also be massaged. Initially, massage here should be for half a minute or so, because any problems will make it tender. However, with further attention it will be possible to work out the soreness. A further point on the leg lies above the knee, in the soft area on the outer edge, above the kneecap. All these reflexes, if worked in turn, will contribute to a healthy system and lead to fewer problems, such as impotence.

Impotence itself can, however, be treated. In addition to

undertaking the massage of reflex points and areas mentioned above, there are further techniques that may help. There is a particularly sensitive and stimulating area between the anus and scrotum, which should be pressed gently a number of times. It is also said that if gentle on-off pressure is applied to the scrotum, this will help.

Another problem faced by many men involves the prostate gland. This gland is situated below the bladder and opens into the urethra, which is the duct carrying urine out of the body and which also forms the ejaculatory duct. On ejaculation, the gland secretes an alkaline fluid into the sperm to help sperm motility. In older men particularly, the prostate gland may have become enlarged, causing problems with urination. Working the appropriate reflexes may help this situation as may massaging the base of the penis. However, it is advisable to check with a medical doctor to ensure that there is no other condition present.

The female reflexes

There are a number of female conditions that may be helped by reflexology. In most cases, the reflexes to be worked are very similar and the following complaints are therefore grouped in this way:

- *amenorrhoea* lack of menstruation, other than during pregnancy or pre-puberty
- *endometriosis* the occurrence of endometrial cells, normally found in the womb, elsewhere in the body, e.g. Fallopian tubes or peritoneum, causing pain and bleeding
- *fibroid* a benign tumour of the uterus that may cause pain, bleeding and urine retention
- *leucorrhoea* discharge of white/yellow mucus from the

vagina, which may be normal before and after menstruation, but at other times large amounts signify an infection
- *dysmenorrhoea* painful menstruation
- *menorrhagia* excessive blood flow during menstruation

For these and related conditions, the general procedure
should be to spend time on the specific female reflex, which
in these cases is the uterus. In addition the endocrine gland
reflexes should be massaged and to provide a balanced treatment, the reflexes for the other reproductive organs (ovary,
etc) should be worked. Further areas to concentrate upon
include the urinary and circulatory systems and the central
nervous system (brain) with the solar plexus.

Premenstrual tension (or syndrome) is the condition typified by headache, nervousness, irritability, depression and
tiredness (in addition to physical symptoms) several days
before the start of menstruation. It is advisable, before menstruation starts, to have a thorough massage of the reflexes
once or twice per week. Next, the reflexes for the uterus and
ovaries should be worked. The uterus reflex is on the inside
of the foot in the soft area beneath the ankle. The massage
should work all around the ankle, beginning with a gentle
pressure, and then working back towards the heel. The other
foot should then be dealt with in the same way.

To help overcome depression the endocrine glands are very
important to regulate hormones, maintain body rhythms and
balance the biochemical functions – all of which have some
effect on emotions. Other reflexes to work, in addition to
the endocrine glands, include the solar plexus, brain and liver.
The liver is very important in this respect and, although the
area should not be overworked, it should not be forgotten.

The *menopause* is the time when a woman's ovaries no

longer release an egg cell every month, and child-bearing is no longer possible. This usually occurs between the ages of 45 and 55. It may be preceded by a gradual decline in the frequency of menstruation or there may be an abrupt cessation. There is an imbalance in the sex hormones and this can cause a number of symptoms, including hot flushes, sweats, palpitations, depression and vaginal dryness. Over a longer period there may be a gradual loss of bone (osteoporosis) leading to a greater risk of bone fractures.

In this instance, the endocrine reflexes are once again very important. In conjunction with these, the reflexes for the spine and brain should be worked, the former to promote relaxation. As a general point, the reflexes to the spine can be massaged for any length of time whereas those for organs and glands should be worked periodically and for a few seconds each time.

To help combat hot flushes, the thyroid reflex should be worked since this is the endocrine gland responsible for the control of the metabolic rate. Regulation of breathing through deep breaths will also help.

The breasts are, of course, the mammary glands that produce milk at the appropriate time, but in today's society they have also become important from a cosmetic point of view. Disorders of the breasts can include lumps or cysts, pain or tenderness. Such conditions may be due to an hormonal imbalance but in any event will benefit from a complete treatment of all the reflexes on feet, hands or head. The breast reflex is found on the top of the foot or hand, at the base of the toes or fingers, and this should be worked regularly. Since the endocrine system is of great significance in the reproductive system, all glands reflexes should receive some attention. Reflexological massage can also be used as a general technique to maintain healthy breasts. Essentially the hand should form a cup around the breast with the fingers underneath and the nipple between thumb and forefinger. Using a circular movement the breast is massaged slightly upwards. This should help retain the shape of the breast, and maintain its tone.

Diseases of the immune system
Antibodies and the lymphatic system
The human body resists infection by means of antibodies and white blood cells. Antibodies are protein substances produced by the lymphoid tissue (spleen, thymus gland and the lymph nodes) that circulate in the blood. They react with their corresponding antigens (foreign bodies that cause antibodies to be formed) and make them harmless. There are a number of immunoglobulins (large protein molecules) that act as antibodies, and each has a particular function. For example, one is responsible for allergic reactions and another is produced to fight bacteria and viruses in the body.

The lymphatic system is also important in the body's immune response. Lymph nodes are swellings that occur at various points in the system. They are found in the neck, groin and armpit, and their main function is to remove foreign particles from the lymph, and to participate in the immune response. In this latter function they become enlarged and produce lymphocytes, a type of white blood cell, which locate and neutralize antigens, or produce antibodies, depending upon their type.

The lymph itself is a colourless, watery fluid. It is derived from blood and is similar to plasma. It contains 95 per cent

243

water, with protein, sugar, salt and lymphocytes. The lymph is circulated by muscular action, and pumped through the lymph nodes for filtering.

It is clear that the lymphatic system, and the immune system overall, are very important in maintaining good health. Any disorder or deficiency in this system will lead to illness, which in some cases may be life-threatening. Reflexology may prove useful in restoring the balance although the need for professional medical advice should always be borne in mind.

Reflex points for the immune system

A number of reflexes to the lymph glands can be worked, on the back of the hands, located over the wrists (*see* the figures on page 203) and on the top of the foot. The spleen is also an important reflex because the spleen itself produces lymphocytes (amongst other things). Associated reflexes that should be worked are those for the endocrine glands, circulation and liver.

In the case of infectious diseases, many of which occur in childhood (such as measles, mumps and chickenpox), the infection will normally run its course and as a result confer immunity to further bouts. To minimize discomfort and aid the recovery, the reflexes for the brain, solar plexus, circulation, endocrine glands and liver should be massaged.

The same applies to most infectious conditions, even autoimmune diseases where the antibodies attack their own body cells. In these cases, the lymph gland reflexes are particularly important.

Shiatsu

Shiatsu, like reflexology, comes from the East. It is an ancient art that works along principles that are very similar to those of acupuncture. Thus it concentrates on the meridians along which the body's energy flows. These meridians must remain clear for the body to function properly. Like acupuncture, shiatsu concentrates on specific points on the body where pressure is applied, but unlike acupuncture, which is very precise and requires years of learning, elements of shiatsu can be practised by people who have a much more basic knowledge than that of the acupuncturist. Shiatsu massage is quite firm and the pressure can be painful at times. It can be given as either as a localized treatment or as a whole-body massage, working along the energy meridians from head to foot.

Origins

Shiatsu originated in China at least 2000 years ago, when the earliest accounts gave the causes of ailments and the remedies that could be effected through a change of diet and way of life. The use of massage and acupuncture was also recommended. The Japanese also practised this massage, after it had been introduced into their country, and it was known as *anma*. The therapy that is known today as *shiatsu* has gradually evolved with time from anma under influences from both East and West. It is only very recently that it has gained recognition and popularity, with people becoming aware of its existence and benefits.

Although East and West have different viewpoints on health and life, these can complement one another. The Eastern belief is of a primary flow of energy throughout the body, which runs along certain channels known as meridians. It is also believed that this energy exists throughout the universe and that all living creatures are dependent upon it as much as on physical nourishment. The energy is known by three similar names, *ki*, *chi* and *prana* in Japan, China and India respectively. (It should be noted that the term 'energy' in this context is not the same as the physical quantity that is measured in joules or calories.) As in acupuncture, there are certain pressure points on the meridians that relate to certain organs, and these points are known as *tsubos*.

The applications of shiatsu

Shiatsu can be used to treat a variety of minor problems such as insomnia, headaches, anxiety, back pain, etc. Western medicine may be unable to find a physical cause for a problem, and although some pain relief may be provided, the underlying cause of the problem may not be cured. It is possible that one session of shiatsu will be sufficient to remedy the problem by stimulating the flow of energy along the channels. A regime of exercise (possibly a specific routine) with a change in diet and/or lifestyle may also be recommended. Shiatsu can encourage a general feeling of good health in the whole person, not just in the physical sense. After some study or practice, shiatsu can be performed on friends and relatives. There are many benefits for both the giver and the receiver of shiatsu, both on a physical and spiritual level.

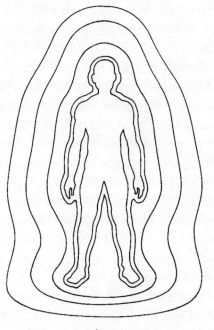

Auras

Energy or ki
Auras
There are believed to be a number of *auras*, or energy layers, that surround the physical body and can be detected or
appreciated (*see* the figure above). The first layer, the *etheric
body*, is the most dense and is connected with the body and
the way it works. An exercise is described later that enables
this layer to be detected. The *astral body* is much wider, is
affected by people's feelings and, if viewed by a clairvoyant, is said to change in colour and shape depending on the
feelings being experienced. The next aura is the *mental body*,
which is involved with the thought processes and intelligence

of a person. Similarly, this can be viewed by a clairvoyant and is said to contain 'pictures' of ideas emanating from the person. These first three auras comprise the personality of a person. The last aura is known as the *causal body*, *soul* or *higher self*. This is concerned more with perceptive feelings and comprehension. It is believed in reincarnation that the first three auras die with the body, but the causal body carries on in its process of development by adopting another personality. As a person grows in maturity and awareness, these different auras are used, and energy is passed from one layer to another. It therefore follows that any alteration in the physical state will, in turn, affect the other layers, and vice versa.

Seven centres of energy, or chakras

It is believed that there are seven main *chakras* (a chakra being a centre of energy) found in a midline down the body, from the top of the head to the bottom of the torso (*see* figure on page 249). They are situated along the *sushumna*, or spiritual channel, which runs from the crown of the head to the base of the trunk. Energy enters the channel from both ends. Since the flow is most efficient when the back is straight, this is the ideal posture for meditation or when powers of concentration are required. Each chakra has a component of each aura, and it comprises what is known as a centre of consciousness. Each aura is activated as a person develops, and the same occurs with the chakras, beginning with the lowest (the *base* or *root chakra*) and progressing to the others with time. There is also a change of energy between the *auras* of each chakra.

The *crown chakra* is concerned with the pineal gland, which

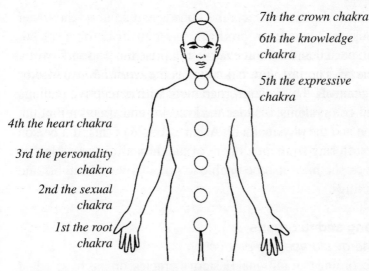

7th the crown chakra

6th the knowledge chakra

5th the expressive chakra

4th the heart chakra

3rd the personality chakra

2nd the sexual chakra

1st the root chakra

The Seven Major Chakras

controls the right eye and upper brain and affects spiritual matters. The *ajna, brow or forehead chakra* also known as *the Third Eye*, is linked with the pituitary gland, which controls the left eye, lower brain, nose and nervous system. It has an effect on the intellect, perception, intuition and comprehension. The *throat* or *expressive chakra* is concerned with the thyroid gland and governs the lymphatic system, hands, arms, shoulders, mouth, vocal cords, lungs and throat. It affects communication, creativity and self-expression. The *heart chakra* is concerned with the thymus gland and controls the heart, breasts, vagus nerve and circulatory system, and affects self-awareness, love, humanitarian acts and compassion. The *solar plexus* or *personality chakra* is concerned with the pancreas. It controls the spleen, gall bladder, liver and digestive system and stomach, and has an effect on desire, personal power and the origin of emotions. The *sacral* or *sexual chakra* affects the gonads and controls the lower back, feet, legs and reproductive system. This affects physical, sexual and mental energy, relationships and self-worth. The *base* or *root chakra* is concerned with the adrenal glands. It controls the skeleton, parasympathetic and sympathetic nervous systems, bladder and kidneys, and affects reproduction and the physical will. As an example of this, if a person is suffering from an ailment of the throat, it is possible that he or she may also be unable to voice private thoughts and feelings.

Zang and fu organs
Energy storage and production
According to traditional Eastern therapies, organs have a dual function – their physical one and another that is concerned with the use of energy and might be termed an 'energetic function'. The twelve organs mentioned in the traditional therapies are split into two groups known as *zang* and *fu*, and each is described below.

Zang organs are for energy storage, and the fu organs produce energy from sustenance and drink and also control excretion. The organs can be listed in pairs, each zang matched by a fu with a similar function. Although the pancreas is not specifically mentioned, it is usually included with the spleen. The same applies to the 'triple heater' or 'triple burner', which is connected with the solar plexus, lower abdomen and the thorax. The lungs are a zang organ and are concerned with assimilation of energy, or ki, from the air, which with energy from food ensures the complete body is fed and that mental alertness and a positive attitude are maintained. This is paired with the fu organ of the large intestine, which takes sustenance from the small intestine, absorbs necessary liquids and excretes waste material via the faeces. It is also concerned with self-confidence. The spleen is a zang organ and changes energy or ki from food into energy that is needed by the body. It is concerned with the mental functions of concentration, thinking and analysing. This is paired with the fu organ of the stomach, which prepares food so that nutrients can be extracted and also any energy, or ki, can be taken. It also provides 'food for thought'. The zang organ of the heart assists blood formation from ki and controls the flow of blood and the blood vessels. It is where the mind is housed and therefore affects awareness, belief, long-term memory and feelings. This is paired with the fu organ of the small intestine, which divides food into necessary and unnecessary parts, the latter passing to the large intestine. It is also concerned with the making of decisions. The kidneys are a zang organ and they produce basic energy, or ki, for the other five paired organs and also for reproduction, birth, development and maturity. They also sustain the skeleton and brain and provide willpower and 'get up and go'. They are paired with the fu organ of the bladder, which stores waste fluids until they are passed as urine and also gives strength or courage. The zang organ of the 'heart governor' is concerned with the flow of blood throughout the body. It is a protector and help for the heart and has a bearing on relationships with other people (although there is no organ known as the 'heart governor' it is connected with the heart and its functions). This is paired with the 'triple heater' or 'burner', which passes ki around the body and allows an emotional exchange with others. The liver is the sixth zang organ, and it assists with a regular flow of ki to achieve the most favourable physiological effects and emotional calmness. Positive feelings, humour, planning and creativity are also connected with it. The gall bladder is the sixth fu organ, with which the liver is paired, and this keeps bile from the liver and passes it to the intestines. It concerns decision-making and forward thinking.

The meridian system

The meridians, as previously mentioned, are a system of invisible channels on the back and front of the body along which energy, or ki, flows. There are twelve principal meridians plus two additional ones, which are called *the governing vessel* and the *conception* or *directing vessel*. Each meridian passes partly through the body and partly along the skin, joining various chakras and organs (the organs as recognized in traditional Eastern medicine). One end of every

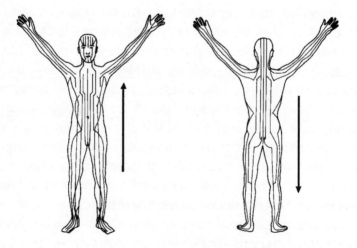

Flow of energy along the meridians

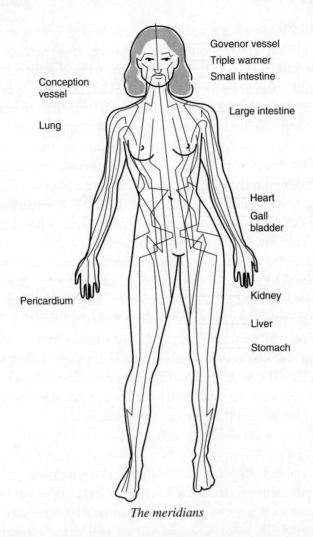

Govenor vessel
Triple warmer
Small intestine

Conception
vessel

Large intestine

Lung

Heart
Gall
bladder

Pericardium

Kidney

Liver

Stomach

The meridians

meridian is beneath the skin while the other is on the surface
of the skin on the feet or hands. Along each meridian are
acupressure or acupuncture points, which in shiatsu are called
tsubos. These points allow the flow of energy along the me-

ridian to be altered if necessary (*see* the figures on pages 252 and 253). The meridians receive energy from the chakras and organs (as described previously), from the meridians with ends located on the feet and hands and also via the pressure points, or tsubos. Energy, or ki, can pass from one meridian into another as there is a 'pathway' linking each meridian to two others. The energy passes in a continuous cycle or flow and in a set order from one meridian to another. By working on the meridians, and particularly the pressure points, a number of beneficial effects can be achieved with problems such as muscle tension, backache and headache. Since the flow of energy is stimulated by working on the meridians this will in turn affect the joints, muscles and skin and thereby ease these complaints. Since a person's mental state, feelings and moods are also altered by the flow of energy, this can induce a more positive frame of mind.

A person in good health should have a constant flow of ki, with no concentrations or imbalances in any part of the body. It is believed that the greater the amount of ki there is within a person's body, the greater the vitality, mental alertness and overall awareness that person will possess.

Feeling ki

It is possible for a person to 'feel' ki, and the following exercise helps demonstrate what it is like. Stand upright with the feet apart and the arms stretched upwards. Rub the hands together as if they were very cold, so that a feeling of warmth is generated. The backs of the hands, wrists and forearms should also be rubbed. The arms should be put down at the side of the body and shaken vigorously. This should then be repeated from the beginning, with the arms above the head and concluding

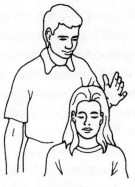

Feeling ki

with the shaking. Then hold the hands out to the front – they should have a pleasant feeling of warmth and vitality, which is due to the circulation of blood and energy that has been generated. The hands should be placed to the sides, then after inhaling deeply concentrate on relaxing as you exhale. This procedure should be done several times, and then it should be possible to feel the ki. The hands should be placed about 1 m (3 feet) apart, with the palms of the hands facing inwards. After relaxation, concentrate your thoughts on the gap between your hands and then gradually reduce the space between them – but they must not touch. It is likely that when the hands come quite close, about 15–30 cm (6–12 inches), a feeling of tingling or warmth may be felt, or the sensation that there is something between the hands. This will be when the auras that surround the hands touch. To reinforce the sensation, the hands should be taken apart again and then closed together so that the feeling is experienced again and becomes more familiar.

The following exercise also enables ki to be felt, but this time it is the etheric aura around another person's head and shoulders. The previous procedure to generate ki should be repeated, but this time the hand should be placed near to another person's head, within 60 centimetres–1 metre (2–3 feet). This person should be sitting upright on the floor or on a chair. The hand should be moved gradually nearer to the seated person's head, concentrating attention on the gap between your hand and his or her head. If no sensation is felt, the hand should be moved back to its original position and the process should be repeated. Again, a feeling of tingling or warmth will probably be experienced as the person's aura is felt. When this has been achieved, the hand can progress round the head and down to the shoulders, noting the edge of the aura at the same time. If the person has no success in experiencing the aura, it is likely that the mind is not clear of other thoughts, so relaxation is suggested prior to any further attempt.

It is also possible for a person, by concentrating his or her thoughts and by a slight change of position, to alter the flow of ki in the body. This will have the effect of either making him or her feel a lot heavier or lighter, depending on which is desired. Taken to extremes, someone who is skilled at the control of ki will prove too heavy to be lifted by four people.

Basic rules

There are some basic rules that should be followed before the practice of shiatsu. Clothing should be comfortable, loose-fitting and made of natural fibres since this will help with the flow of energy or ki. The room should be warm, quiet, have adequate space and be neat and clean. If not, this can have an adverse effect on the flow of ki. The person receiving the therapy should ideally lie on a futon (a quilted Japanese mattress) or similar mat on the floor. If necessary, pillows or cushions should be ready to hand if the person does not feel comfortable. Shiatsu should not be given or received by someone who has just eaten a large meal – it is advisable to delay for several hours. No pressure should be exerted on varicose veins or injuries such as cuts or breaks in bones. Although shiatsu can be of benefit to women while pregnant, there are four areas that should be avoided and these are the stomach, any part of the legs from the knees downwards, the fleshy web of skin between the forefinger and thumb, and an area on the shoulders at each side of the neck. Ensure that the person is calm and relaxed. It is generally not advisable to practise shiatsu on people who have serious illnesses such as heart disorders, multiple sclerosis or cancer. An experienced practitioner may be able to help, but a detailed and accurate diagnosis and course of treatment is essential. A verbal check on the person's overall health is important and also to ascertain if a woman is pregnant. If there is any worry or doubt about proceeding, then the safest option is not to go ahead.

Although the general feeling after receiving shiatsu is one of wellbeing and relaxation, there are occasionally unpleasant results, such as coughing, generation of mucus or symptoms of a cold; a feeling of tiredness; a headache or other pains and aches; or feeling emotional. The coughing and production of mucus is due to the body being encouraged to rid itself of its surplus foods (such as sugars and fats) in this form. A cold can sometimes develop when the mucus is produced, usually when the cells of the body are not healthy. Tiredness can occur, frequently with a person who suffers from nervous tension. After therapy has removed this stress or tension, then the body's need for sleep and rest becomes apparent. A short-lived headache or other pain may also develop, for which there are two main reasons. Since shiatsu redresses the balance of ki in the body, this means that blockages in the flow of energy are released and the ki can rush around the body, causing a temporary imbalance in one part and resulting in an ache or pain. It is also possible that too much time or pressure may have been applied to a particular area. The amount needed varies considerably from one person to another. If a pain or headache is still present after a few days, however, it is sensible to obtain qualified medical help. Emotional feelings can occur while the energy is being stimulated to flow and balance is regained. The feelings may be connected with something from the past that has been suppressed and so, when these emotions resurface, it is best for them to be expressed in a way that is beneficial, such as crying. There may, of course, be no reaction at all. Some people are completely 'out of touch' with their bodies and are aware only that all is not well when pain is felt. If this is so, then any beneficial effects from shiatsu may not register. Because of a modern diet that contains an abundance of animal fats, people become overweight through the deposition of fat below the skin and around the internal organs. The body is unable to 'burn off' this fat, and this layer forms a barrier to ki. The flow is stopped, and overweight people do not tend to benefit as much because of the difficulty in stimulating the flow of ki in the body.

Exercises and the three main centres

The body is divided into three main centres – the *head*, the *heart*, and the *abdominal* centres. The head centre is concerned with activities of a mental nature, such as imaginative and intellectual thought processes, and is concerned with the brow chakra. The heart centre is concerned with interactions among people and to the world in general, including the natural world. It is related to the chakra of the throat and heart. The abdominal centre is related to the base, sacral and solar plexus chakras and is concerned with the practical aspects of life and physical activity. Ideally, energy should be divided equally among the three but because of a number of factors, such as activity, education, diet, culture, etc, this is frequently not so. In shiatsu, more importance is attached to the abdominal centre, known as the *hara*. The following exercise uses abdominal breathing and, by so doing, not only is oxygen inhaled but also ki is taken into the hara where it increases a person's vitality. Once the technique is mastered, it can be practised virtually anywhere and will restore composure and calmness.

Sit on the floor with the back straight and, if possible, in the position known in Japan as *seiza* (*see* figure below). The hands should be placed loosely together in the lap and the

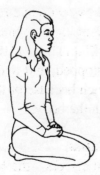

Seiza

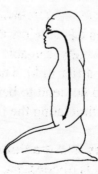

Inhaling through the nose

mind and body should become relaxed after some deep breathing. One hand should be put on the stomach, below the navel, and the other on the chest. When inhaling, this should not be done with the chest but with the abdomen, which should increase in size. As the person exhales the abdomen should contract, and this procedure should be practised for a few minutes. After a rest it should be repeated, inhaling quite deeply but still the chest should not be allowed to rise. Some people may not find this exercise at all difficult while others may need more practice. It may be that there is stress or tension in the diaphragm. Once the technique has been mastered and the hands do not need to be placed on the chest and abdomen, imagine that ki is being inhaled down into the hara. Sit in the same position and inhale slowly via the nose and imagine the ki descending (*see* figure on page 259). (It may aid concentration if the eyes are closed.) The breath should be held for about four seconds and concentration should be centred on the ki. Then exhale gradually through the mouth and repeat the process for a few minutes.

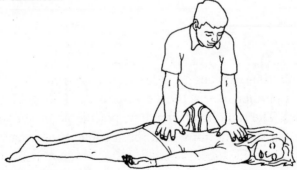

A centred movement

The next exercise is known as a centred movement, which practises movement of the ki, since it is one person's ki that should have an effect on another. After practising shiatsu on a partner, you should not feel tired but refreshed and exhilarated. This is a benefit of the extra ki in the body. The exercise should be begun on hands and knees (a body width apart), and it is most important that you are relaxed and comfortable with no tension. This position is the basis for other movements that are practised on others. While the position is maintained, begin to move the body backwards and forwards so that you are conscious of the transfer of weight, either on to the hands or knees. The body should then be moved slowly in a circular way, again being aware of the shift of weight from the hands, to hands and knees, to knees, etc, returning to the original position. You should also realize that as the whole body is moved, the abdomen is its 'centre of gravity'. Practise maintaining a position for about five seconds, registering the increase in weight on the hands when you move forwards and the reduction when you rock backwards. Then return to the original position. It is important that the body weight is always used at right angles to the receiver as this will have the maximum effect on the flow of ki. The reason for holding a particular position is that this has the effect of making the person's ki move.

The centred movement previously described can be practised on a partner in exactly the same way, following the same rules. The right hand should be placed on the sacrum, which is between the hips, and the left hand midway between the shoulder blades. As before, you should rock forwards and hold the position for about five seconds and then repeat after rocking backwards on to the knees (*see* figure above). This basic procedure can be repeated about twelve times, and if you are not sure whether too much or too little pressure is being used, check with your partner. You will eventually acquire the skill of knowing what amount is right for a particular person.

To summarize, there are some basic rules to be followed when practising shiatsu. A person should make use of body weight and not muscular strength, and there should be no effort involved. At all times a calm and relaxed state should be maintained, and the weight of the body should be at right angles in relation to the receiver's body. The person's whole body should be moved when altering weight on to the receiver, maintaining the hara as the centre. Any weight or pressure held should be for a short time only and both hands should be used equally. It is best to maintain a regular pattern of movement while giving shiatsu, and always keep in physical contact with the receiver by keeping a hand on him or her throughout the therapy.

Shiatsu on the face and head

There are a large number of different exercises and techniques, but at each time the giver must be relaxed and calm to enable the flow of ki to occur and thus make the shiatsu work to full effect. As an example, the following exercise on the face and head begins with the receiver's head being held firmly in one hand and, using the thumb of the other hand, pressing upwards in a straight line between the eyebrows towards the hairline. Each movement should only be quite small, about 12 millimetres (0.5 inch). The fingers should then be placed on each side of the head and both thumbs used to press from the inner end of the eyebrows

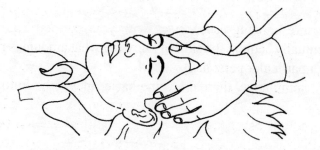

A – Press between the eyebrows towards the hairline

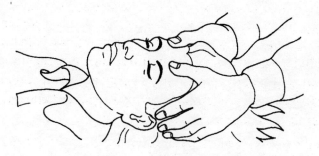

B – Press from the eyebrows across the brow

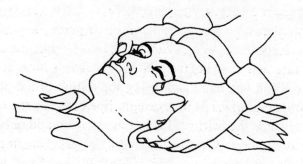

C – Work the thumbs across the bone below the eyes

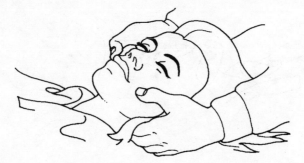

D – Press across the face below the cheekbones

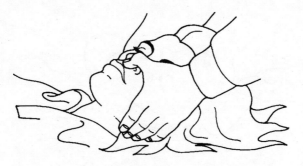

E – Press the area between the nose and upper lip

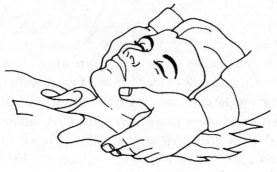

F – Press with the thumbs outwards over the upper jaw

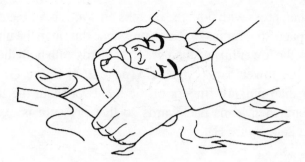

G – Outwards over the lower part of the jaw

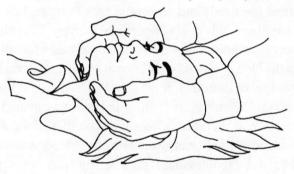

H – Place fingers beneath the jaw and lean back

towards the hairline (*see* page 263, figure A). Again, holding the hands at each side of the head, the thumbs should then be used to press from the start of the eyebrows across the brow to the outside (page 263, figure B). With the fingers in place at each side of the face, work the thumbs across the bone below the eyes, moving approximately 6 millimetres (0.25 inch) at a time (page 263, figure C). Commencing with the thumbs a little to one side of each nostril, press across the face below the cheekbones (figure D). Press one thumb in the area between the top lip and nose (figure E) and then press with both the thumbs outwards over the upper jaw (page 264, figure F). Next, press one thumb in the hollow below the lower lip and then press outwards with both thumbs over the lower part of the jaw (page 264, figure G). The giver then puts all fingers of the hands beneath the lower jaw and then leans backwards so that pressure is exerted (page 264, figure H).

Kyo and jitsu energy

As a person progresses in the study of shiatsu and comes to understand the needs and requirements of others, he or she will gradually be able to give beneficial therapy. It is believed that energy, as previously defined, is the basis for all life, and it is divided into two types known as *kyo* and *jitsu*. If the energy is low or deficient, it is known as kyo, and if there is an excess or the energy is high, it is known as jitsu. These two factors will therefore affect the type of shiatsu that is given and, with practice, it should be possible to assess visually and also by touch what type a person is. A few general guidelines as to how a person can vary his or her shiatsu to suit either kyo or jitsu types are given below. As the person progresses, however, it is likely that an intuitive awareness will develop of what is most suitable for a particular person. For kyo types (low or deficient in energy), a gentle and sensitive touch is required, and any stretched positions can be maintained for a longer time as this will bring more energy to that part of the body. Pressure, held by the thumb or palm, can also be maintained for an increased length of time, approximately 10–15 seconds. For jitsu types (high or excess energy), the stretches can be done quite quickly so that the energy is dispersed, and also shaking or rocking areas of the body can have the same effect. The pressure that is exerted by the thumbs or palms should also be held for a shorter length of time, so that excess energy is dispelled.

Yin and yang

As previously mentioned, a change in diet may also be recommended by a shiatsu practitioner. From the viewpoint of traditional Oriental medicine, food can be defined in an 'energetic' way. This differs from the Western definition of foods consisting of protein, minerals, fats, carbohydrates, fibre and vitamins. It is believed that, according to its 'energetic' definition, food will have differing physical, mental, spiritual and emotional effects. This energy is split into two parts known as *yin* and *yang*. Yin is where energy is expanding and yang where it is contracting. They are thus opposites and, from traditional beliefs, it was thought that interactions between them formed all manner of occurrences in nature and the whole of the world and beyond. All definitions of yin and yang are based on macrobiotic food (a diet intended to prolong life, comprised of pure vegetable foods such as brown rice), this being the most usual reference. Food can be divided into three main types – those that are 'balanced', and some that are yin and some that are yang. Foods that are defined as being yin are milk, alcohol, honey, sugar, oil, fruit juices, spices, stimulants, most drugs (such as aspirin, etc), tropical vegetables and fruits, refined foods, and most

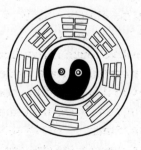

Yin and yang

food additives of a chemical nature. Yang foods are poultry, seafood, eggs, meat, salt, fish, miso and cheese. Balanced foods are seeds, nuts, vegetables, cereal grains, beans, sea vegetables and temperate fruits (such as apples and pears).

The balance between yin and yang is very important to the body, for example, in the production of hormones such as oestrogen and progesterone, and glycogen and insulin and the expansion and contraction of the lungs, etc. A 'balanced' way of eating, mainly from the grains, beans, seeds, nuts and vegetables, etc, is important as this will help to achieve the energy balance in the meridians, organs and chakras, as defined previously. When these two opposing forces of yin and yang are in harmony and balanced, physical and mental health will result.

Body reading

It is possible for practitioners of shiatsu, as they become increasingly experienced, to assess a person's physical and mental state of health by observing the body and forming accurate observations. If the traditional ways of Eastern diagnosis are studied, this can assist greatly. The Eastern methods were based on the senses of hearing, seeing, smelling and touching and also by questioning people to obtain information leading to an overall diagnosis. This is known as body reading.

Makko-ho exercises

Makko-ho exercises are six stretching exercises, each of which affects one pair of the meridians by stimulating its flow of energy. If the complete set of exercises is performed, all the body's meridians will have been stimulated in turn, which should result

in increased vigour and an absence of tiredness. Before beginning the exercises, you should feel calm and relaxed. It may
prove beneficial to perform some abdominal breathing first (as
previously described). One example is the triple heater and heart
governor meridian stretch. Sit on the ground with either the feet
together or crossed. The right hand should grasp the left knee
and the left hand the right knee, both quite firmly (*see* figure A
below). Then inhale and, as you exhale, lean forwards and downwards with the top half of the body so that the knees are pushed
apart (*see* figure B below). Hold this position for approximately
30 seconds while breathing normally, and then, after inhaling,
return to the upright position. After completion of all exercises,
lie flat on the ground for several minutes and relax.

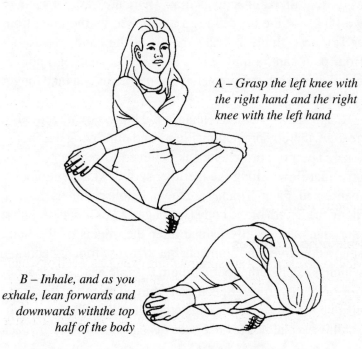

*A – Grasp the left knee with
the right hand and the right
knee with the left hand*

*B – Inhale, and as you
exhale, lean forwards and
downwards withthe top
half of the body*

Acupressure

This is an ancient form of healing combining massage and acupuncture, practised over 3,000 years ago in Japan and China. It was developed into its current form using a system of special massage points and is today still practised widely in the Japanese home environment.

Certain 'pressure points' are located in various parts of the body and these are used by the practitioner by massaging firmly with the thumb or fingertip. These points are the same as those utilized in acupuncture. There are various ways of working and the pressure can be applied by the practitioner's fingers, thumbs, knees, palms of the hand, etc. Relief from pain can be quite rapid at times, depending upon its cause, while other more persistent problems can take longer to improve.

Acupressure is said to enhance the body's own method of healing, thereby preventing illness and improving the energy level. The pressure exerted is believed to regulate the energy that flows along the meridians, qi or ki. As previously mentioned, the meridians are the invisible channels that run along the length of the body (*see* page 253 of Shiatsu). These meridians are mainly named after the organs of the body such as the liver and stomach, but there are four exceptions, which are called the 'pericardium', 'triple heater', 'conception' and 'governor'. Specifically named meridian lines may also be used to treat ailments other than those relating to it.

Ailments claimed to have been treated successfully are back

pain, asthma, digestive problems, insomnia, migraine and circulatory problems, amongst others. Changes in diet, regular exercise and certain self-checking methods may be recommended by your practitioner. It must be borne in mind that some painful symptoms are the onset of serious illness so you should always first consult your G.P.

Before any treatment commences, a patient will be asked details of lifestyle and diet, the pulse rate will be taken along with any relevant past history relating to the current problem. The person will be requested to lie on a mattress on the floor or on a firm table, and comfortable but loose-fitting clothing is best so that the practitioner can work most effectively on the energy channels. No oils are used on the body and there is no equipment. Each session lasts from approximately 30 minutes to 1 hour. Once the pressure is applied, and this can be done in a variety of ways particular to each practitioner, varying sensations may be felt. Some points may feel sore or tender and there may be some discomfort such as a deep pain or coolness. However, it is believed that this form of massage works quickly so that any tenderness soon passes.

The number of treatments will vary from patient to patient, according to how the person responds and what problem or ailment is being treated. Weekly visits may be needed if a specific disorder is being treated while other people may go whenever they feel in need. It is advisable for women who are pregnant to check with their practitioner first since some of the acupressure methods are not recommended during pregnancy. Acupressure can be practised safely at home although it is usually better for one person to perform the massage on another. Common problems such as headache, constipation and toothache can be treated quite simply although there is the possibility of any problem worsening first before an improvement occurs if the pressure points are over stimulated. You should, however, see your doctor if any ailment persists. To treat headache, facial soreness, toothache and menstrual pain, locate the fleshy piece of skin between the thumb and forefinger and squeeze firmly, pressing towards the forefinger. The pressure should be applied for about five minutes and either hand can be used. This point is known as 'large intestine 4'.

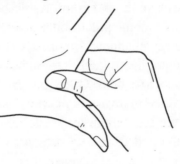

Large intestine 4

To aid digestive problems in both adults and babies, for example to settle infantile colic, the point known as 'stomach 36' is utilized, which is located on the outer side of the leg about 75 mm (3 ins) down from the knee. This point should be quite simple to find as it can often feel slightly tender. It should be pressed quite firmly and strongly for about five to ten minutes with the thumb.

When practising acupressure massage on someone else and before treatment begins, ensure that the person is warm, relaxed, comfortable and wearing loose-fitting clothing and that he or she is lying on a firm mattress or rug on the floor.

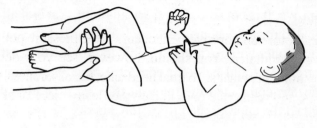

Stomach 36

To discover the areas that need to be worked on, press firmly over the body and see which areas are tender. These tender areas on the body correspond to an organ that is not working correctly. To commence massage using fingertips or thumbs, a pressure of about 4.5 kg (10 lbs) should be exerted. The massage movements should be performed very quickly, about 50 to 100 times every minute, and some discomfort is likely (which will soon pass) but there should be no pain. Particular care should be taken to avoid causing pain on the face, stomach or over any joints. If a baby or young child is being massaged then considerably less pressure should be used. If there is any doubt as to the correct amount, exert a downwards pressure on bathroom scales to ascertain the weight being used. There is no need to hurry from one point to another since approximately 5 to 15 minutes is needed at each point for adults, but only about 30 seconds for babies or young children.

Using the 'self-help' acupressure, massage can be repeated as often as is felt to be necessary with several sessions per hour usually being sufficient for painful conditions that have arisen suddenly. It is possible that as many as 20 sessions may be necessary for persistent conditions causing pain, with

273

greater intervals of time between treatments as matters improve. It is not advisable to try anything that is at all complicated (or to treat an illness such as arthritis) and a trained practitioner will obviously be able to provide the best level of treatment and help. To contact a reputable practitioner who has completed the relevant training it is advisable to contact the appropriate professional body.

Reiki

Reiki is a method of natural healing which is centred upon *universal life energy*, the meaning of the Japanese word *Reiki*. The therapy was named after Dr Mikao Usui, a Japanese theologist, who rediscovered the art of healing using and by transferring this universal life energy. Following a prolonged period of meditation, Dr Usui acquired the ability of transferring Reiki energy. He was also able to help others to act as channels for this energy.

To benefit fully from the technique, you must be initiated into at least the first degree of Reiki. This is done by a Reiki master. The initiation is merely a means whereby the universal life energy is bestowed through the Reiki master. The master acts as a channel and a link to release the healing power.

Reiki energy

Reiki energy is regarded as life energy at its most effective – with the maximum vibration. It is considered to have an almost divine quality and as such includes everything, in a world where problems and disorders are deemed to be due to the feeling of detachment from the world. When a person undergoes a session of therapy, they allow the energy to be taken into themselves with beneficial effects.

Those who use Reiki regularly often find they are more joyful, lively and their own inbuilt energy is enhanced – almost as if their batteries had been fully charged!

The treatment
Effects and limitations

There are several inter-related effects that result from taking in Reiki energy:

- it enables the universal life energy to be received;
- it creates a feeling of deep relaxation;
- energy blockages are removed allowing a flow of life energy throughout the body;
- toxins of various sorts are removed; these and other waste products are removed from the system much more quickly.

When the toxins have been removed from the body, more energy can be received and the vital processes and functions become more highly tuned. When the body takes in more and more life energy, it is said that its frequency becomes higher, facilitating contact with the Universal Spirit and generating trust in the universal life energy.

Deep relaxation is central to Reiki therapy and this is very much dependent upon the divine quality attributed to the energy. The extent to which Reiki can work is defined by the receiver of the energy because only the necessary amount of energy is drawn in. If the receiver is not accepting of the energy or feels negative about it then its effectiveness will be restricted

Whole-body Reiki
Preparation

Reiki is best applied to the whole body, to cleanse and revitalize the complete system.

Many practitioners undertake a particular routine before commencing a regime of whole-body treatment and the main elements are briefly described below.

Jewellery should be removed asit has the potential to create interference in the reception of the Reiki energy.

The hands should be washed because the aura (see page 247) surrounding the body may be affected by contact with objects, people, etc over the course of the day and washing removes such influences.

It is helpful at this stage to recite a short prayer asking for healing and to concentrate upon and acknowledge your aims.

Even out the aura

This is a means of starting the therapy:

- the subject should lie down (*see* figure below)
- sitting at his or her side put your left hand on your sacrum
- with your right hand held about 15–25 cm (6–9 inches) above the body and palm facing down, move your hand along the length of the body from the head to the toes
- return the hand to the starting point using a circular motion along the side of the body
- repeat this three or four times

This process can be repeated after the Reiki when your left hand can be placed on the sacrum of the healee.

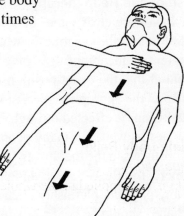

Energize

When each Reiki therapy session is complete the whole body may be energized via the root chakra (*see* page 249).

Even out the aura

The hand is held vertically above the body and then quickly moved from the pelvis to the head.

Before the treatment

There is great scope for variation in the number and sequence of positions used for whole-body treatment. The extent of each session of Reiki will vary depending upon circumstances and the individual receiving treatment. Certain positions may be better left out of the sequence or therapy may be focussed on a particular area to help relieve blockages or deal with tension.

If dealing with a small child or an elderly or infirm person, it is probably wise to limit the therapy to a session of 15 to 20 minutes. In all cases the Reiki practitioner should be sensitive to and aware of the condition, needs and well-being of the recipient.

Positions in Reiki therapy

The hands are clearly the 'instruments' of healing in Reiki and although the position in which they are placed on the recipient is meaningful, it may not be possible, nor is it essential that the exact position is copied. Just placing the hands on the appropriate part of the body will suffice.

Reiki can be effected through clothing, as the energy will flow just as well, but many people prefer to have no material obstacles to the therapy. In this case, and particularly for partners, the Reiki can be undertaken in the nude. If there are any physical blemishes such as a burn or other wound, the hands should be held a few inches above the skin at this area, around the corresponding acupuncture point, or reflex zone.

The head

On the *head*, the basic position is shown in the figure below. The hands are placed either side of the nose, with the palms covering the eyes; the thumbs rest by the bridge of the nose and the fingertips cover the cheeks and reach the upper lip. This arrangement covers the sinuses, eyes, pituitary gland, teeth and is useful for dealing with colds, sinusitis, eye complaints, allergies, fatigue and general discontent.

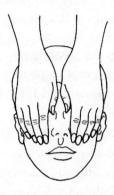

The basic position for the head

In the second arrangement for the head, the hands are placed over the ears, with the fingertips extending down the jawline to the neck, encompassing the ears of course which includes the semi-circular canals, responsible for balance. The effect also extends to the pharyngeal area. Diseases and problems of these organs – colds, trouble with balance, hearing loss, etc – are dealt with in this arrangement.

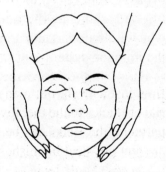

*Alternative arrangement
for the head*

279

If the hands are placed on the back of the head, this helps with conditions such as headaches, colds, asthma and circulatory problems. It generally promotes relaxation.

The chest and abdomen
The next sequence of hand arrangements is for the chest and abdomen. Once again there are many variations, but a selection is presented here.

The arrangement for the thymus, heart and lungs is as follows: one hand is laid across the thymus and the other is at 90° starting just below and between the breasts. The thymus is a bilobed gland in the neck which is an important part of the immune system. This arrangement therefore reinforces the immune system and helps the lymphatics, the heart, lungs and counters any general debility.

The next illustration in the sequence shows the hands placed either side of the na-

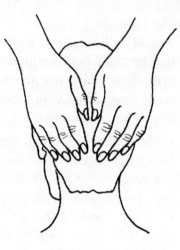

Position for hands on the back of the head

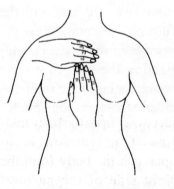

Arrangement for thymus heart and lungs

vel and slightly to one side. The stomach and digestive organs are the focus of attention here and the conditions/symptoms addressed necessarily have a link with these body systems. As such this will help digestion and the metabolism in general terms, and specifically will combat nausea, heartburn, gastrointestinal diseases and indigestion. Because the presence of such conditions often results in tension and worry, the relief of symptoms will similarly help relieve anxiety and depression.

Next are two positions in which the hands are placed in a position similar to that shown in the arrangement used to focus on the stomach and digestive organs but further away from the body midline. One version is to approach the body from the right side of the partner/client. The left hand is placed around the base of the ribcage and in this way the gall

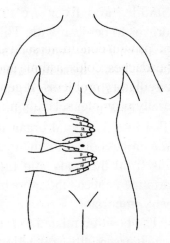

Arrangement for stomach and digestive organs

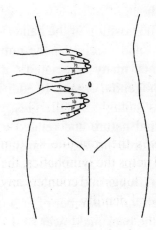

Arrangement for the gall bladder and liver

bladder and liver are the organs to be dealt with. This position is for diseases and conditions of these important organs and associated problems of a metabolic nature. The liver is a vital organ in the process of removing toxins from the body and this arrangement can therefore be very important.

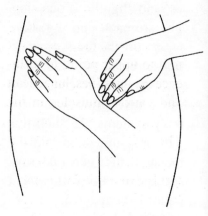

Arrangement for the appendix intestines and urogenital organs

The position related to this one is essentially a reflection, where the hands are placed on the left side of the body to encompass the area of the bowels, spleen and some of the pancreas. Accordingly diseases of these organs, indigestion and healthy blood are all dealt with.

The position of the hands where the pelvic bones are covered and meet over the pubic area is for a number of ailments, many associated with the appendix, intestines and urinogenital organs. In addition, this arrangement is considered suitable for allergies, general debility, problems of a sexual nature and related to weight and is appropriate to reinforce the immune system.

The back

There are a number of arrangements which can be adopted on the back and lower back. The figure shows one such position with a number of effects but it is likely that by gently experimenting, a slightly different yet equally beneficial arrangement can be found. Here the hands are placed across the shoulder blades at mid to upper point, to influence the intestines, lung, heart and various muscles in the neck and shoulder region. This will help lung and heart diseases, muscular tension, headaches and related conditions.

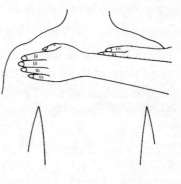

Focus on the back to help lungs, heart, muscular tension and headaches

If the hands are placed lower down the back, around the midriff (on the lower ribs) this position will accommodate the kidneys and adrenal glands. (The adrenal glands are situated one each on the upper surface of each kidney and are important because they manufacture hormones that control a variety of body functions, e.g. adrenaline is one hormone produced).

In addition to these specific positions, there are many other Reiki positions to deal with a multitude of complaints and the reader is referred to a more extensive account for greater detail. It

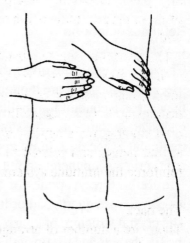

Focus on the lower back to help kidneys and adrenal glands

must always be remembered that serious conditions or diseases of a particular nature should be dealt with by the appropriate specialist.

Reduction of side-effects
In the case of many drugs, uncomfortable, distressing and even threatening side-effects can ensue. Reiki can be a very useful adjunct for anyone taking a course of drugs. It can help reduce some side effects and generally aid the body in recovery when the course has been completed. Post-operative recovery will benefit from Reiki and it can also help after chemotherapy. In all these cases Reiki therapy supplies that extra life energy, enabling the body to bounce back more quickly from the burdens of surgery and chemicals.

In some cases, use of Reiki therapy after an operation may lessen pain and the natural healing processes will be accelerated.

Reiki associations
Crystals
Crystal therapy is involves the use of precious and semi-precious stones that are thought to hold positive energy and they act as a conduit for healing from the practitioner to the recipient. In some cases the stone is placed on the body where treatment is focused, in others it may be positioned on the appropriate acupuncture point.

In Reiki, three varieties of quartz are commonly used – amethyst, rose quartz and ordinary quartz (or rock crystal). The crystal structure of quartz is often taken to be related to the six chakras and the tip of the crystal to the seventh chakra. Practitioners recommend using rock crystal to avoid feeling overpowered by changes, mounting pressures and the stress of everyday life. Carrying the crystal or wearing it is meant to bring light into your workaday routines.

Meditation

Meditation needs concentration and time and a will to continue with the practice. Some of the benefits may happen straight away (such as a lowering of the blood pressure) while others require some proficiency.

Reiki assists in this concentration. There are some positions that can be adopted in Reiki meditation to achieve particular goals. In the first position the legs are drawn up and the soles of the feet put together with the knees falling apart. This can be done while lying down or sitting against a wall. The hands adopt a praying gesture. The Reiki energy removes any blockages and performed regularly, this becomes a powerful meditation exercise.

Aromatherapy

When used in conjunction with Reiki, some oils can be applied directly on particular areas of the body, or their aroma can be made to fill the room using an aroma lamp. Below a few oils are considered and their use compared to their therapeutic value in aromatherapy. It is very likely that someone with a knowledge of essential oils will be able to capitalize upon their experience and incorporate further oils in their Reiki therapy.

- *Lavender* – In Reiki, lavender is associated primarily with patients/recipients who are sensitive and easily hurt, essentially introverts. It can be used in long sessions of Reiki when the lavender helps to promote the calm and confidence necessary for a period of building and strengthening of the life force energy.

- *Sandalwood* – Produces an ambience conducive to Reiki because the oil is considered to elicit trust and confidence, between practitioner and recipient.
- *Clary sage* – In a session of Reiki, clary sage has been used to open blocked channels and to enhance sensitivity.
- *Patchouli* – Patchouli is used in Reiki therapy to enhance the sensual qualities and aspects of life.

Prescription drugs

Reiki makes the body more receptive and therefore therapy prior to a course of drugs may enhance the effect of the drug. The relaxed state engendered by Reiki may, however, counter, to some extent, the efficacy of an anaesthetic.

Although minor pains can often be remedied through the use of Reiki alone, stronger pain killers do not have their effect lessened by Reiki. The interaction between Reiki and drugs is neither well tested nor documented, but the overall positive effect of the therapy means that it is not likely to cause any problems.

Homoeopathy

In conjunction with this therapy, Reiki provides a reinforcing effect by rendering the treatment more effective. Reiki can help avoid strain, improve the removal of toxins and increase the body's sensitivity.

Bach remedies

These are named after Edward Bach, an English doctor, who in the early years of this century gave up his Harley Street practice to concentrate upon finding plants with healing qualities. He identified 38 plants, the flowers of which he floated on clear spring water. This, he believed, transferred medicinal properties to the water which could be given to patients. This practice he developed to mimic the drops of dew on the plant which in the first instance were used. Intended for home self-help, the remedies are meant for treating the whole person. Stock solutions are diluted in water and a few drops taken.

Typical examples are:

- cherry plum for fear, tension, irrationality
- holly for envy, jealousy and hatred
- pine for guilt and constantly apologizing
- sweet chestnut for despair
- wild rose for apathy

In common with many other examples, Reiki improves the effectiveness of Bach remedies.

Chakras

A chakra is a centre of energy in Reiki. In addition to being 'representative' of a particular organ or group of organs, a chakra also controls our being on different levels and it links these two representative states.

In Reiki there is considered to be seven major and a number of minor chakras. The seven major chakras are shown in the figure on page 249.

The root chakra is the source of strength and is essential for proper development. Disorders within the root chakras may result in mental problems.

The sexual chakra governs sensual and sexual factors. Blockages result in conditions such as a fear of being touched. Physical manifestations may include problems with the kidneys/bladder or lymphatic system.

The personality chakra, also called the solar plexus chakra, is the power centre and focus of personal freedom or, conversely, feelings of guilt. Consequences of a blockage might be anxiety about how others perceive you, envy or selfish greed. Physically there could be digestive disorders.

The heart chakra controls self-acceptance. Blockages may result in attitudes such as selfishness. Physical manifestations could be disorders of the lungs and heart, and circulatory problems.

The expressive chakra, or throat chakra, controls self-expression. An upset in this centre could well result in an individual who becomes dictatorial. Physical signs could be growth problems, or lack of vocal control.

The knowledge chakra, forehead chakra or Third Eye, is the focus of intuition. A blockage will culminate in a haphazard approach to life, and probably an inability to settle down to any one task for any length of time.

The crown chakra is generally felt that the seventh, crown, chakra is appreciated only by experience and it depends upon the other six for its development.

Conclusion

Reiki is a technique of healing available to anyone. It can lead to a more relaxed approach to life and greater harmony with the total environment. It can also be applied to plants and animals, for example your household pets, and for this and further information about the therapy, the reader is advised to seek more detailed treatments.